· THE MYSTERIOUS BRAIN ·

THE WORLD'S OLDEST INFORMATION PROCESSOR

Director Brain Research Advocates
Information Network (B.R.A.I.N.)

Salvatore Amoroso

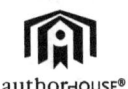

authorHOUSE®

AuthorHouse™
1663 Liberty Drive, Suite 200
Bloomington, IN 47403
www.authorhouse.com
Phone: 1-800-839-8640

First published by AuthorHouse 5/22/2008

ISBN: 978-1-4343-8474-4 (sc)

Printed in the United States of America
Bloomington, Indiana

This book is printed on acid-free paper.

CONTENTS

INTRODUCTION

The title of this book is based on the fact that most of how the brain works is still a mystery. The three pound jelly-like mass of tissue squeezed inside our skulls is by far the most complex and least understood organ of the human body. It has even been described as the most complex living structure known in the universe. Most researchers agree that there is more we do not know about the brain than we do know in order to completely understand how the brain works. This presents a significant and urgent scientific challenge, considering that the brain is the source of all human actions and interactions, both positive and negative. It is not too far-fetched to say that the future of the world depends in large part on the human brain. Understanding how it works will help us to learn who we are and how we can lead more satisfying and productive lives. This makes brain science (neuroscience) an important present and future field of study and research. As we continue to unlock the present mysteries of the brain we will not only find cures and preventions of brain diseases and mental illnesses, but we will learn more about ourselves as human beings. This new knowledge will change the course of human history.

The brain falls in the category of an information processor, in the sense that it accepts input data (the five senses), performs analyses of the data, and provides outputs.

The subtitle of this book refers to the human brain as the "worlds oldest information processor", which technically is incorrect, since all animal brains are information processors as well, and they have been around in various forms for millions of years. But the human brain as we know it today is certainly the oldest processor of its kind, with capabilities that are truly remarkable. The human brain has been around for at least 250,000 years, belonging to the species called "homo sapiens". Although the size and probably the architecture of the brain has probably remained the same over that period of time, the tasks performed have changed significantly. The brain has showed tremendous ability to adapt to change, and to grow in capability.

Thinking of the brain as an information processor will surely make learning about the brain more interesting to today's computer-smart younger generation. Information technology (IT) is advancing at such a rapid pace, that one wonders where it will take us. The personal computer has certainly helped propel both the information revolution, and the digital revolution. Analog electronic information processing preceded the digital revolution, but solid-state electronics technology and digital (binary) signal processing have rapidly found widespread application. The creative capabilities of the human brain seem to be almost limitless.

It could be argued that information technology began when humans perfected the techniques of language, beginning with the spoken word, and followed by the written word. This progression has grown into electronic communications, including radio and television, both of which preceded the digital revolution, which arrived along with the first personal computers in the 1970's. Digital (binary) coding of information (data) is highly compatible with solid-state technology, and provides important signal-to-noise advantages. Interestingly, the million or so year old brain design uses a form of digital signal processing, and like the computer, performs all of its magical processing with a very small number of basic circuit components. This is not to say that either the computer or the brain are simple or easy to understand processors. They are very complex. Analogies between the brain and the computer do exist, but the differences are far greater than the similarities. Furthermore, the computer still has a long way to go before it will be able to out-think the human brain.

During this information technology revolution, it is surprising that the world's oldest and to date most capable information processor, the human brain, has not been given much attention by information technology scientists. This is unfortunate from the point of view of brain science, which advances relatively slowly in the medical research community, where learning how the brain works is secondary to finding new drug treatments for brain disorders. New drugs can mean huge profits for companies, whereas new information about how the brain works cannot be patented and is therefore of far less interest.

It is my strong belief that brain research (neuroscience) needs to be elevated to a much higher priority by our government agencies involved in basic scientific research. And by higher priority I also mean that adequate funding needs to be made available. It is meaningless to declare a "Decade of the Brain" at even the presidential level, as did George W. Bush in 1990, if it is not backed up by funding and specific project goals. We do exactly that with respect to exploration of "outer space". We need to do the same with respect to exploring "inner space", namely the human brain. It is the information processor called the human brain that will largely determine the future of the human species. It seems logical to me that learning more about how the brain works will result in being able to maximize its performance, as well as providing the best treatments for brain disorders, and ultimately preventative measures. Knowing more about how the brain works will result in improved educational methods. The field of "brain-based" education has already begun based on what we know about the brain already, which is certainly a lot. But most brain researchers admit we have a long way to go. Some say we only know about 10% of what we need to know. Even if the number is 50%, the need for research is undeniable.

My objective in the following pages will be to discuss what we now know about the brain, based on my review of the literature, and then to identify the remaining unknowns that will challenge dedicated scientists for well into the future. The level of technical detail will be for the person or student with limited understanding of the brain, but who wants to get an exposure to the field of neuroscience. An excellent introductory book about the brain, titled "Brain Facts" is available from the Society for Neuroscience (www.sfn.org) free of charge, and I recommend it highly. Neuroscience will be of interest and benefit to children of all ages as well as adults.

One of the most important reasons for the average person to learn more about the brain is to enable us to make better decisions with respect to our mental healthcare. In a recent report by the National Institute of Mental Health, it was stated that 50% of Americans will personally experience a serious mental illness episode at least once in their lifetime. Those who assume that it will not happen to them, or if it does, they will rely on some miracle medication to cure the problem, are deluding themselves. Medical science has not progressed as far in the treatment of mental illness as it might seem from the drug advertisements. Many of the drugs used to treat mental illnesses have potentially serious side effects, and some can be addictive. In any case, an educated consumer is in the best position to help make treatment decisions. Even an elementary knowledge of what we already know about how the brain works will reveal that the present "chemical imbalance" theory of brain disorders is a far too general and over-simplified explanation for mental illnesses.

My research for writing this book has included a lot of excellent books, by recognized experts on the subject of the brain (see bibliography), but many of them tended to be overly technical for the average person. I have also made use of the internet and medical journals for exploring the state-of- the-art in neuroscience. As in most areas of science, the amount of information available is enormous. Much of the material was way over my level of understanding, and tended to be narrowly focused in a single technical area. I have tried to combine and condense this material into a relatively short book that might be useful as a guide for an introductory course on the subject of the brain. The subject is important enough, in my opinion, for there to be elementary, middle and high school versions of brain science courses. But we first need to get educators themselves interested in learning more about the brain and how it works, so they can be motivated to teach their students. After all, learning about how we learn is one of the key challenges being addressed by brain science, and this should be of fundamental interest to educators. There is already a lot of material being marketed under the topic of brain-based education, and it is important for educators to be able to evaluate this new information.

We will never know for sure who designed the human brain, but it may be within our power to eventually learn how it works. Let's explore what scientists presently do and do not know about how the brain performs its magic.

EXPLORING INNER SPACE

Before beginning our exploration of the human brain, or inner space, as it could be called, let's first consider the two words "brain" and "mind". Is the word "mind" just an alternative for the word "brain", or is there a real difference, either scientifically or otherwise? I have read elaborate descriptions by various authors of how the mind is something beyond the brain. To me, none of the arguments are very convincing. We can probably all agree that the human brain is the biological organ that resides within the skull. The word "mind" could arguably be simply an alternate terminology for the living, active brain. Certain phrases in our language would not sound right if we didn't continue to use both words, regardless of their meanings, for example, saying "my mind is made up" would sound strange as "my brain is made up". The important thing is to learn how the brain works as opposed to what we call it. We need not get side-tracked by non-scientific explanations of mind/brain differences. If and when we understand completely how the brain works, the mind/brain questions will be answered as well.

One simple way to think of the mind is to consider it to be the word that refers to the functioning brain in a living human being. An autopsied brain in a jar is clearly no longer a mind. Historically, the organ called the brain has not commanded the kind of respect it deserves, for example, as compared to the relatively simple pump called the heart. Past history has afforded the heart far more powers than it actually exhibits. The arts are full of references to the human heart that rightfully belong to the brain. This is technically not a problem for the arts, since its purpose is to entertain and not to educate. But it is about time for the brain to take its rightful place as the central processing unit of the human organism, a processor that can do things that computers will likely never come close to doing, and the source of all human creativity. The word brain is being used more and more in everyday life by both the media and educators, and this is a good thing. The brain needs to be de-mystified if we are to take maximum advantage of what science knows about the brain, now and in the future.

My own personal interest in brain science partly derives from my 30 year career as an electrical engineer designing state-of-the-art radar and communications systems. My career spanned both the analog and digital signal processing eras. The signal processing that goes on in the brain is similar in some basic ways to that which we design engineers did in our systems, at least in terms of electrical operation. The brain, however, is also a complex chemical based processor, and the combination has produced what we now know as the human brain.

The worldwide scientific effort to "map the human genome" is an example of successful goal-oriented science. Now we need an effort to "map the human brain". Learning how the brain works will be a process of "reverse engineering" that will require scientists of many different specialties working together towards that common goal. Clearly this is no easy task. The brain is by far the most complex organ in the human body, and the most difficult to access for measurement and experimentation. But the potential payoff is too great not to have a national program at least equivalent to our exploration of outer space.

The good news is that a lot of basic research is going on, both with government and private funding. Much progress is being made in understanding how the brain works, and we can see from books being sold and from television documentaries that the average person , especially children, are anxious to learn about their "central processing units". Hopefully this trend will encourage capable students to pursue careers in science, and particularly neuroscience. We as a nation have the resources, if we keep our priorities in order, to explore both "outer space" and "inner space".

Interestingly, although the reasons for exploring both realms are similar, the technological tools are very different. Outer space exploration obviously involves very large distances, whereas inner space exploration involves the exact opposite. In brain science we are forced to look at microscopic and eventually probably sub-microscopic levels to get answers. A simple mathematical way to look at it is that one science aims towards (+) infinity and the other towards (-) infinity. Both explorations have immense potential for benefits, but in my opinion brain science is even more important than the science of outer space.

Before too long, it is likely that engineers will design electronic devices that will be able to probe the internal workings of the living human cell, and build electronic interfaces between living cells and mechanical devices which will revolutionize medicine, biology and electronics. However, if we want the United States to continue to be the leader in these important technological areas, we need to make science more attractive to students. This will be no easy task for a society that seems obsessed with the fields of entertainment, sports, and business.

The inner-space world of microscopic activity may not seem to have the excitement and glamour of the world of space-ships and astronauts. But clearly the future of the human race is heavily dependent on learning more about this molecular and even sub-molecular space that we will call inner-space. When scientists entered the atomic and sub-atomic world, they found that the classical physical principles of the larger world did not adequately explain the atomic level world. A new field of physics, called quantum mechanics, has developed within the last century to study matter and radiation at an atomic level. A detailed explanation of quantum mechanics is well beyond the scope of this book, but it is interesting to know that such a scientific field exists to study the fundamental reality of matter, including the matter of life. The world can be divided into the familiar realm that we perceive, obeying classical laws, and the invisible quantum world which exhibits a curious mixture of wave and particle characteristics. A detailed scientific understanding of both worlds will be required before all of the brain's mysteries will be revealed.

Neuroscience is the official name for the field of brain research, but I prefer to call it brain science. "Neuro" is the Greek word for "nerve" and is also the source of the word neuron, which is sometimes called the brain cell, or the nerve cell. In this case I prefer the term "neuron" since they are present in both the brain and the nervous system..

NEURONS, SYNAPSES AND SIGNAL PROCESSING

Weighing only about three pounds and fitting within the skull, the brain is certainly the most complex organ of the body. Some scientists have described the brain as the most complex device in the known universe. Science has already revealed much about the composition and functioning of the brain, but much remains to be learned. Surprisingly, all of the brain's functions are made possible by specialized cells called neurons together with their interconnecting elements called dendrites, axons, and synapses.. The complexity comes in the numbers of these components, their operation and their interconnections, much of which remains unknown.

The basic building block of all living things are "cells", which typically contain an organized complex of biological molecules, including DNA, surrounded by a plasma membrane. Cells are very small, usually measuring between 10 to 100 micrometers across. The brain's electrical signals are generated by charged atoms, called ions, that are present both inside and outside the cell membrane, in particular, positively charged sodium and potassium ions, and negatively charged chloride atoms. In the resting state, the inside of a brain cell has a net negative charge relative to the outside of the membrane.

There are many different types of specialized cells in the body, but the brain contains two basic cell types, namely "neurons" and "glia". The neurons handle all of the signal processing that goes on in the brain, using a combination of both electrical and chemical processes. The glia cells provide a variety of support functions for the neurons, but are not involved with signal transmission. It is estimated that the brain has upwards of 100 billion neurons, and probably 10 times that number of glia cells. The glia cells may have functions that we do not yet understand. The basic building blocks of all the brain's circuitry are neurons, dendrites, axons, and synapses What the brain lacks in variety of building block elements, it certainly makes up in quantity of those it does have.

Neurons have the unique ability to grow filaments called dendrites and axons, which allow it to communicate with other neurons. A membrane covers the axons and dendrites as well as the cell body. The space outside the membrane is called the extra cellular space and is filled with a variety of chemicals, some with electrical charges, that influence cellular function. The axons are cell output channels, dendrites are input channels. These nerve fibers conduct electricity, but in a special way. Electricity does not flow passively through a neuron and its fibers as it does through a wire. Rather impulses conducted through nerve fibers are biologically propagated, moved along by electrochemical actions, a process that takes a lot longer than passive physical conduction. The biologically propagated impulse generated by the neuron is called an "action potential", which is an electrical pulse that travels down axons at a speed of about 200mph, which may seem fast, but in fact is very slow compared to electricity flowing in a wire (conductor) which travels at the speed of light (186,000 mph).

The connection between neurons is made by a very important element called a "synapse". The synapse is a very tiny gap (approximately one millionth of a centimeter) between the axon of a sending neuron and the dendrite of the receiving neuron. The synapse has a valve-like property which means that transmission is in only one direction. It also has a threshold type characteristic, requiring some minimum amount of neurotransmitter reception before allowing re-transmission of an electrical pulse. Researchers have learned that there are both electrical and chemical type synapses, but that the dominant form of synapse transmission is chemical. The interconnection of pre-synaptic and post-synaptic cells is shown in Figure 2(a). The basic structure of the chemical synapse is shown in Figure 2(b). The neurotransmitter chemicals are usually produced and stored in sacks (vesicles) at the synapse. Once enough of the neurotransmitter molecules are received at the post-synaptic receptors, a smaller version of the action potential called a "post-synaptic potential (psp)" results which travels via the dendrite to the receiving neuron. Thus much of what the brain does involves electrical-to-chemical-to-electrical conversions of signal information.

One-way transmission between neurons results from the fact that synaptic transmission involves the release of chemicals from storage sites in the pre-synaptic axon terminal. These molecules are released when action potentials from the cell body reach the terminal. The released chemicals then drift across the liquid-filled synaptic space and come in contact with dendrites or other portions of the post-synaptic cell. Because the chemical storage sites are in the pre-synaptic terminal and the receptors are in the post-synaptic dendrite, transmission occurs in one direction only. The chemicals are called neurotransmitters, since they allow neurons to communicate across the synaptic gap- they "transmit" between neurons.

Most neurons have only one axon, however, each axon branches many times before it ends, allowing a single neuron to communicate with many others. Many dendrites have little knobs extending from them called spines, and each spine can make a synaptic connection with axons from other neurons. Some axons are covered with a substance called myelin (see Fig 2a). This myelin sheath, as it is called, has gaps in it that allow the action potential impulse to propagate, since the ion gates that generate the impulse are only present in the gap areas. In effect, the impulse jumps from gap to gap resulting in faster propagation in myelin covered axons. This speed is important in the central nervous system where axons can be relatively long.

Neurons can be either "projection", also called "excitatory", type neurons, whose role it is to turn on the next projection cell in the circuit, or "inhibitory" type, whose role is to prevent generation of an action potential in the post-synaptic cell, The inhibitory neurons can thereby regulate the signal traffic through a given area, and probably de-activate areas of the brain when we sleep. With the 100 billion or so neurons to work with, the brain is able to be wired in a lot of different ways. Before birth, our genes basically control the wiring process, but after birth it appears that both genes and experience effect the connection configuration. Experience (learning) works by modifying the "expression of genes", which in turn re-configures the brain. Electron microscope photographs of interconnected neurons in the brain are shown in Figures 2(c) and (d), from the "Brain Mania" C-D from The Brain Store (www.thebrainstore.com.).

SIGNAL PROCESSING AND NEURAL NETWORKS

Neurons in effect add up a set of quantities (dendrite inputs), compare the sum to a threshold, and indicate whether the threshold is exceeded. With correct weightings of the dendrite inputs, the three basic logic gate configurations of digital computers can be implemented with neurons. The first description of a neuron as a "basic threshold unit" was made in a 1943 paper by McCulloch and Pitts. Threshold units are very simple models of neurons, which can be interpreted as simple logic machines (Fig. 2e). The basic threshold unit computes its activation as the sum of its (positive) excitation and of its (negative) inhibition coming from the active input cells. If the activation is larger than some established threshold level, then the unit fires, which corresponds to transmitting an output level of one (1). If the activation is smaller than the threshold, then the output value of the cell is zero (0). Thus the response of the threshold unit depends upon its level of activation, which is computed as the sum of the weighted inputs from active input cells. With correct weightings of the dendrite inputs, the basic logic gate configurations of digital computers can be implemented with neurons.

The study of neuronal (or neural) circuitry and networks has been ongoing for many years. When large numbers of neuron-like elements are connected into networks, mathematicians have been able to construct signal processors that are able to perform brain-like functions. But the brain has not yet been mapped to the point where actual circuit or network configurations can be defined. The simplest type of neural networks are called feed-forward networks whose goal is to "learn" some association between input and output patterns. A detailed discussion of neural networks is well beyond the scope of this book and is a scientific field of its own. Interestingly, engineers have all but ignored the neural network approach to systems, in favor of the digital (binary) design approach. Only time will tell how far the digital "revolution" will take us, but we know it has a long way to go in producing a system like the human brain.

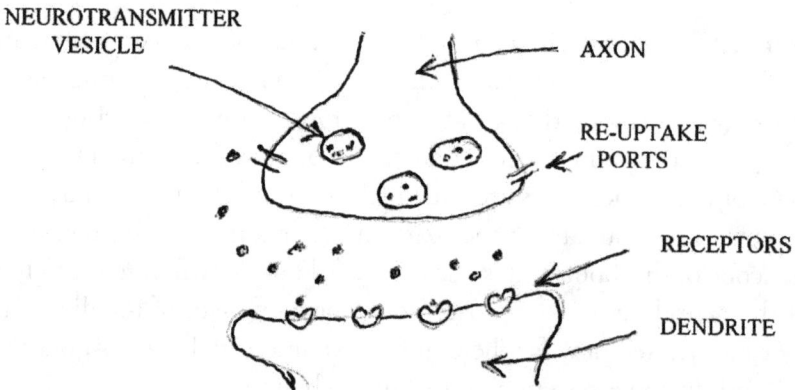

INPUTS

CELL BODY

MYELIN
SHEATH

DENDRITES

SYNAPSES

AXON

OUTPUTS

FIGURE 2 (a)   NEURON (BRAIN CELL)

NEUROTRANSMITTER
VESICLE

AXON

RE-UPTAKE
PORTS

RECEPTORS

DENDRITE

FIGURE 2 (b)   SYNAPSE

The Neuron Jungle

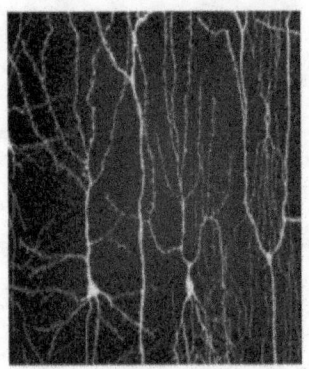 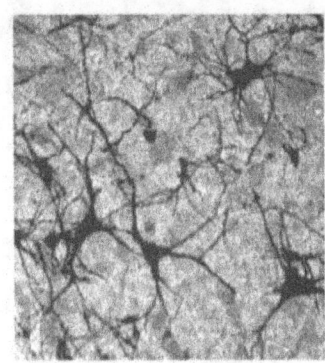

In different areas of the brain, there are distinctly different patterns of neurons, but there is always complexity and wonder.

Figure 2C

The Neuron Jungle

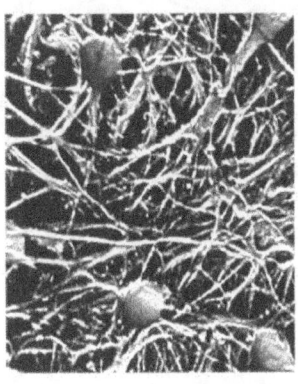 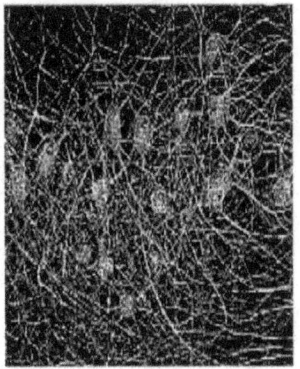

At increasing magnification, we see the extraordinary density and intertwining of the brain's billions of neurons.

Figure 2D

FIGURE 2 (e)   BASIC THRESHOLD UNIT

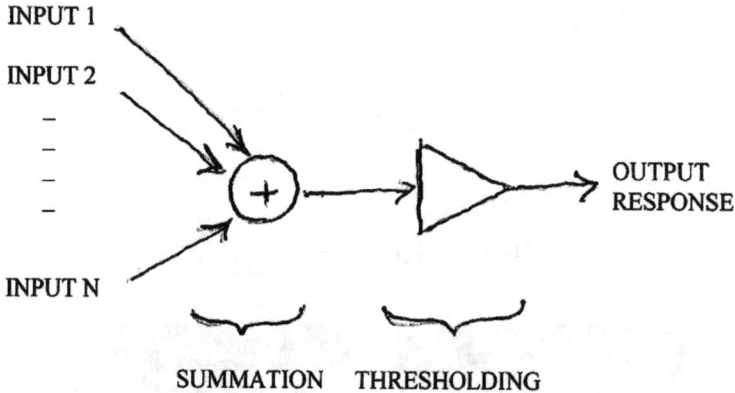

3

ARCHITECTURE
AND FUNCTIONS

In computer terminology, the brain could be called the central processing unit (CPU) of the overall human body. Analogies between computers and the brain are interesting and useful for understanding what we know about how the brain works. But the fact is that the brain is very different from present day computers. Most importantly, the brain can think, reason, and generate new ideas, things that computers may never be able to do. The architecture of the brain is basically fixed by design, however, certain functions such as learning and memory are clearly programmable throughout life.

The brain is bio-electrical, bio-chemical, and even bio-mechanical, whereas the computer uses primarily solid-state technology. Computers use binary digital signal processing and a common timing "clock" for synchronization. The brain is not a pure analog or digital signal processor, and uses a form of variable frequency, pulse-coded signal format. The brain appears to have many specialized processors working in parallel, with no apparent timing or synchronizing means. One of the major advantages of the computer's digital or "binary" format, which has only two distinct signal levels (on/off or 1/0) is noise immunity (low-level extraneous signals). This is a very important characteristic for any information processor, and indeed the brain's neurons also provide a noise reducing "threshold" effect, in generating their action potentials. Computers have a single master "clock" which dictates the timing of all the serially performed data processing steps. This has the useful side effect of preventing system overload. Unfortunately, our brains seem to be more subject to information processing overload. But it is amazing how resilient the human brain actually is, considering all of the use and abuse that it is subjected to over a lifetime.

In computers, the "software" is clearly distinct from the "hardware", whereas in the brain the picture is not as clear. But it is not unreasonable to say that the brain is "programmable" by both genetic and environmental (learning) processes. In brain science terminology, the brain, including the adult brain, has "plasticity", which means that it can grow new neurons and change wiring configurations. Cognitive therapy, which is the alternative to drug therapy for treatment of certain mental disorders, is based on the fact that the brain is re-programmable to some degree. The field of cognitive therapy will be advanced as scientists learn more about how the brain works.

The brain is one overall complex assembly, but it does have a number of identifiable structures having separate functions, with names assigned by medical researchers over the past several hundred years. On the internet website of the Harvard Medical School, there is a list called the 100 Brain Structures (actually 106). One can click on each named structure and view an MRI scan showing the location in the brain. Personally, I think that 100 parts may be applicable for medical students, but is too many for most of the rest of us. My preference is to start off thinking about the brain architecture in three major parts, which can be called **1) THE COGNITIVE CENTER, 2) THE EMOTIONAL CENTER, and 3) PRIMITIVE CENTER.**

The COGNITIVE CENTER corresponds to what is usually called the CEREBRUM and is the site of most conscious (voluntary) and intellectual activities. This is the part of the brain which separates us from the rest of the animal world. The EMOTIONAL CENTER is commonly called the LIMBIC SYSTEM and is comprised of several structures within the physical center of the brain. The components of this system and their interconnections contain most of the elements that define individual personality, cognitive style, and patterns of behavior. THE PRIMITIVE CENTER which includes the Cerebellum and Brainstem are responsible for most of the automatic and life-sustaining activities.

Within the three defined major sections of the brain are eleven important sub-structures (or modules) that are commonly mentioned in the literature. Table I is a listing of these modules and a brief summary of their probable functions.

TABLE 1.......THREE PART MODEL OF THE BRAIN
(and major modules)

I. **COGNITIVE CENTER** (Cerebrum- left and right hemispheres)
       A. FRONTAL LOBES (behind forehead)
    Intellectual functioning
    Thought processes
    Behavior and decision-making
    Language- Comprehension and generating speech
      B. PARIETAL LOBES (top of brain-contains sensory and motor cortex)
    Controls muscles of opposite side of body
    Analysis of sensations
    Processes sense of touch
     C. TEMPORAL LOBES (lower sides of brain)
    Hearing and understanding speech
     D. OCCIPITAL LOBES (lower rear of brain)
    Vision processing

II. **EMOTIONAL CENTER** (limbic system)
- A. AMYGDALA
  - Receives all sensory inputs
  - Fear and emotions
  - Captures traumatic memories
  - Regulates sleep
- B. HIPPOCAMPUS
  - Memory formation
  - Turns off the stress response
- C. HYPOTHALAMUS
  - Controls endocrine (hormonal) system and stress response
  - Regulates temperature
  - Regulates sleep, sexual behavior, mood, and emotions

- D. THALAMUS
  - Initial processor for sensory inputs (except smell)
  - Initiates responses for extreme of temp and pain

III. **PRIMITIVE CENTER** (brainstem/cerebellum)
- A. CEREBELLUM
  - Coordinates motor activity
  - Storage of primitive reactions and learned programs that have become automatic
  - Balance, posture, and coordinated movement
- B. MEDULLA
  - Controls automatic activities of heartbeat, breathing, blood pressure and digestion
- C. PONS
  - Receives information from facial skin, eyes, nose and mouth
  - Controls jaw, eye, and muscles for facial expressions
  - Controls saliva and tears

At adulthood, the brain makes up only about 2% of the body's weight, but consumes about 20% of the body's energy. The CEREBRUM comprises almost 80% of the overall brain. The CEREBRUM is usually defined as consisting of two halves called the left and right CEREBRAL HEMISPHERES. The thin outer dense layer of the cerebral hemispheres is called the CEREBRAL CORTEX (or just CORTEX). It is the size and functioning of this portion of the brain that sets humans apart from all other animals. It gives us the unique abilities to "think" and to "reason", as opposed to mostly just following instincts and reacting to the environment. The left and right hemispheres of the brain are interconnected by a large bundle of nerves called the CORPUS CALLOSUM. For some reason, women have more connections in the corpus callosum than men! Another somewhat surprising characteristic of the brain's architecture is that the right hemisphere controls the left side of the body and the left hemisphere controls the right side of the body. Scientists tell us that for 90% of people language resides in the left hemisphere, for 5% in the right hemisphere and for the remaining 5% it is split between hemispheres.

The literature usually describes each hemisphere of the cerebrum as being divided into four sections, or lobes, as follows; the FRONTAL LOBES, the PARIETAL LOBES, the TEMPORAL LOBES and the OCCIPITAL LOBES. The occipital is in the back and is where the visual cortex is located. The frontal lobe, obviously, is in the front, and rests just above the eyes on each side. Between the occipital and frontal lobes are the parietal and temporal lobes. The parietal lobe sits of top, and the temporal lobe is just below it, right behind and slightly above your eyes.

It is useful to consider brain sections for discussion purposes, but in reality the vast number of interconnections between sections makes the real brain look more like one single, but very complex overall system. The characterization of left-brain/right-brain is commonly discussed, and in fact there is a physical divide between the left and right parts of the cortex (cerebral hemispheres). But as discussed in the last paragraph, the two halves are connected by a bundle of about two million separate wires (corpus callosum), which means there is considerable cross-communication going on. Inter-communication seems to be a basic characteristic of the brain's architecture. Figures 3 (a), (b), (c), and (d) show views of the brain that depict make-up and function location. These pictures are also from the "Brain Mania" C-D.

We are characterizing the brain as an information processor, but its architecture and functioning is very different from the typical computer. It is evident that the brain does a lot of processing simultaneously (in parallel), which makes it more powerful and fast reacting. Computers are very structured by comparison, and performs its signal processing in a serial, step-by-step process under control of a master timing "clock". When electrical engineers design complex overall systems they usually start with a simplified overall "block diagram" to describe the inputs, outputs, and major functional elements that comprise the system. My version of a simplified block diagram of the brain is shown in Figure 3 (e).

The basic signal INPUTS to the brain are the five senses, namely sight, sound, smell, taste, and touch, plus signals from inside the body for regulation of various functions. There is a massive amount of information contained in the sensory inputs, so that the brain's initial function is to decide what to use and what to ignore. The brain processes the sensory inputs such that we are able to see, hear, smell, taste, and feel. Scientists know a lot about the brain's components and circuitry involved in these processes, but exactly how all this electro-chemical signal processing results in our overall consciousness and being "alive" is still beyond explanation, and is one of the foremost mysteries of life.

The brain is bathed inside and out by cerebro-spinal fluid (CSF) that contains nutrients (glucose, proteins, and salts) and byproducts of brain activity. The regions inside the brain containing CSF are called ventricles. The brain itself is protected by three layers of membrane coverings called MENINGES within the skull. CSF circulates within two of these layers and this configuration helps protect the brain against shocks.

The brain is kept alive by a continuous flow of blood from the circle of arteries fed by the carotid arteries, which run up each side of the front of the neck and from two vertebral arteries that run parallel to the spinal cord. The brain receives about 20% (1/5) of the blood pumped by the heart, and if deprived of blood (oxygen) for 2 or 3 minutes, or glucose for 10 or 15 minutes, serious brain damage could result.

The membrane surrounding the brain also serves as a protective filtering mechanism, called the blood-brain barrier, protecting the brain from some poisons and unwanted chemicals that are in the blood. STROKES are serious events affecting the flow of blood to the brain. Blockages of blood flow are either caused by a blood clot (CEREBRAL THROMBOSIS) or by material that comes from elsewhere in the body (CEREBRAL EMBOLISM). Less common, but most serious form of stroke is called a CEREBRAL HEMORRHAGE, which is a rupture of a blood vessel and bleeding within or over the surface of the brain.

Considering the harsh environment in which it operates, the brain and its enclosure are very well designed, but apparently intended for some limited amount of lifetime. The theoretical maximum lifetime for a human organism is still unknown, but it should continue to increase as medical science advances.

The brain is definitely an information processor. It accepts inputs, processes them, and provides outputs. A summary of these elements is listed as follows:

BRAIN INPUTS- THE FIVE SENSES

Sensory inputs to the brain arrive from different types of receptors (sensors) for each of the five senses, but all of them supply electrical signals compatible with the brain's signal processing circuitry. The sensory receptors are each uniquely sensitive to one type of input, and have the ability to generate electrical impulses when activated. In the field of electrical engineering, sensors (usually called transducers) are commonly used to interface a system with the real world, and include microphones, keyboards, motion sensors, and a very long list of other types.

All of the brain's sensory inputs (except smell) enter by way of the brainstem and midbrain, and then to the thalamus, which is a small round structure located at the very center of the brain. Some amount of processing of the sensory inputs are performed in these locations before the information is relayed to the higher cognitive centers of the brain for further analysis and possibly memory. One purpose of this initial processing is apparently to allow us to almost reflexively direct us to orient towards the specific stimuli. Information based on the five senses are not all processed in the same area of the brain, probably because they require different types of processing. But somehow all this information is integrated in some way so that we can experience all of our senses together.

The signal processing architecture of the brain seems consistent with the fact that it is a product of evolution, with the brainstem and midbrain structures being one of the earliest forms in animals that processed the same input stimuli that humans process. It is logical for the original sensory signal pathways to have remained the same, as more complex brains formed, culminating in the human brain of today. One can only wonder what the next step will be in the evolution of the brain.

The sensory receptors are sometimes called selective transducers, because they convert the energy contained in the stimulus to another form of energy. The energy contained in the stimulus is used by the receptor to change the conductance of its membrane for one or more ions which results in the generation of an action potential which is sent to the brain via specific bundles of nerves (axons). Since action potentials are fixed amplitude impulses, they do not convey information as to the intensity (strength) of the input stimulus. To convey this intensity parameter, the sensory neurons have the ability to vary the repetition rate (frequency) of the action potential. A very wide dynamic range of stimulus strength can be represented because of the logarithmic relationship between stimulus strength and action potential frequency. On a logarithmic scale, the output changes an equal amount for every 10 to 1 change in the input. Receptors can thereby linearly encode variations of input intensity of about 11 orders of magnitude (110 decibels) which is a very large dynamic range.

Receptors are divided into 5 major types based on the input stimulus to which they are most sensitive. They are;

1) Chemoreceptors- respond to chemical molecules that bind to the receptor.

2) Mechanoreceptors- respond to various forms of mechanical energy such as pressure and vibration.

3) Thermoreceptors- respond to temperature.

4) Photoreceptors- respond to light.

5) Nociceptors- respond to noxious, painful stimuli.

VISION

The eye's retina acts as a photo-transducer to convert light into action potentials that travel to the brain via the optic nerves. The retina contains about 125 million receptors composed of 2 types called "rods" and "cones". Rods are most sensitive to dim light and do not convey the sense of color. Cones work in bright light and are responsible for acute detail, black and white, and color vision. There are three types of cones that are sensitive to red, green, and blue light which in combination convey information about all the visible colors. The retina consists of four layers. The back layer called the pigmented layer is the last one to receive light and absorbs light to prevent it from reflecting back to the forward layers. The next layer contains the rods and cones, and above the rods and cones we have what is called the bipolar cell layer which collects the information from the rods and cones and passes it to the fourth layer called the ganglionic layer. Ganglionic cells have extensions which gather together to form the optic nerve. Light passes through the first two layers before reaching the rods and cones.

The retina has roughly 120 million rods, 6 million cones, and 1 million ganglion cells. Cones are concentrated in the central region of the retina. The central most point of this area, where we focus images most sharply is called the fovea, which contains only cones and no rods. The ratio of cones to bipolar cells to ganglion cells is 1:1:1 which allows this region to send vast amounts of data to the brain and thereby provide high resolution vision. As we move farther out from the fovea, a greater number of rods and cones interact with each bipolar cell and more bipolar cells interact with each ganglionic cell, such that resolution is decreased. About 100 rods communicate with each bipolar neuron, and about 5 bipolar neurons communicate with each ganglionic neuron in the region of the rods. So the information from the rods is lower in resolution than the information from the cones. However, the rod area has high light sensitivity and therefore provides improved night vision.

Each eye sends information via its individual optic nerve to a common location called the optic chiasm where some of the fibers cross and some do not. The optic nerves contain about one million axons. The optic tracks then lead to the thalamus which brings together information from both eyes. From the thalamus the information is passed on to the visual cortex in the occipital lobe of the cerebrum. It is believed that different aspects of vision, such as shape, color, location and motion recognition are processed separately in different cortical areas. Exactly how the astronomical numbers of action potentials are processed and result in our being able to "see" is still a subject for study by scientists.

SOUND

Sound waves enter the ear and cause the eardrum to vibrate and pass the vibration onto the middle ear and then to the inner ear, which has a fluid filled structure called the cochlea. The inner ear is also involved with balance, and contains a structure consisting of three semicircular canals (tunnels) filled with liquid. At the end of each canal is a small swelling covered with receptor cells shaped like tiny hairs, the bending of which produces electrical signal, which are sent to the brainstem which is responsible for maintaining physical balance. Inside the cochlea are the sensors that convert sound-wave vibrations into electrical signals. The sensors are hair-like projections attached to a membrane called the basilar membrane (sometimes called the labyrinth). The membrane is like a very thick skin and divides the cochlea (spiral shaped tube) lengthwise. There are about 16,000 hair-cell sensors in each ear that connect to 28,000 fibers in the auditory nerve that carries the information to the brain. Sounds are represented by both amplitude (loudness) and pitch (frequency). A very large dynamic range of sound intensities can be heard due to the logarithmic compression characteristic of some sensors such as the hair-cells, as discussed earlier. Different sound frequencies maximally activate different hair cells down the cochlea because of fluid movement differences based on the cochlea shape. High frequencies activate hair cells at the beginning of the cochlea, middle frequencies about midway down the length, and low frequencies at the inner most tip of the cochlea spiral. Auditory nerves enter the brainstem where some processing takes place and then via the thalamus to the auditory cortex of the temporal lobe. Initial processing in the brainstem results in positioning of the head and adjusting of the pressure in the inner ear to optimize reception of sounds. Speech sounds, however, are probably processed differently from others. When speech sound is perceived the neural signals are sent to the left hemisphere for processing in language centers.

TASTE

Receptors (taste buds) on our tongue measure the presence of four primary tastes (sweet, salty, sour and bitter). The taste receptors undergo a constant replacement cycle over a period of about 10 days. Each taste bud consists of about 100 sensory cells (receptors). We have about 9000 taste buds in and around the mouth, including the tongue, cheeks, roof of the mouth, and in the throat. This means that the average person has upwards of one million taste sensors. For taste buds to be activated, the detected chemicals must be dissolved in the saliva (as opposed to airborne for smell receptors). The taste buds are also directly connected to salivary glands which contain salivary cells that produce saliva. The sensations of taste and smell are closely linked as evidenced by food's lack of taste when our noses are blocked. The pathway for taste information is via the brainstem to the thalamus and then to the cortex.

SMELL (Olfactory System)

Receptors located in a small patch of mucus membrane lining the roof of the nose detect chemical information in the air we inhale, as well as what is shunted upward from the mouth as we chew our food. The olfactory membrane is approximately 1 inch square and contains almost 100 million total smell receptors. There appear to be four basic smells that we can differentiate: fragrant (like roses), fresh (like pine), spicy (like cinnamon), and putrid (like rotten eggs). Different proportions of the basic smells can be combined to create a large number of recognizable smells. Some persons can apparently discern thousands of odors. The portion of the sensory cell that is exposed to odors posses hair-like cilia. The cilia contain the receptor sites that are stimulated by odors carried by airborne molecules. Olfactory receptors undergo a constant cycle of replacement about every 30 days. The information about smells is sent to the amygdala and to the olfactory cortex. The direct route traveled by olfactory information to the amygdala is a holdover from early evolution, when quick emotional responses to odors played a crucial role in survival.

TOUCH (including pressure, temperature, pain)

Receptors sensitive to touch are located throughout the body and send signals via the spinal cord and brainstem to the thalamus and somatosensory cortex (parietal lobe). Touch is the first of the 5 senses to develop and is considered a key component in growing, learning, communicating and living. In hairy skin areas, some receptors consist of webs of sensory nerve cell endings wrapped around the hair bulbs. They are very sensitive and are triggered when the hair moves. Other receptors in the non-hairy areas consist of nerve cell endings that may be free or surrounded by bulb-like structures. Various parts of the body have different touch resolution, for example in the fingers it is high (1/10 inch) whereas in the thighs it is low (3 inches). Human skin is sensitive to vibrations in the frequency range of about 5-500 hz. Pain messages about tissue damage are picked up by special receptors called "nociceptors". Some pain responses such as reflex responses can occur without brain processing. Most signals are transmitted to the spinal cord and then to the brainstem, thalamus, and cerebral cortex. These pain messages can be suppressed by a system of neurons that originate in the midbrain (at the top of the brainstem) and have a descending pathway down the spinal cord where the pain signal can be suppressed. Some of these descending pathways use naturally-occurring opiate-like chemicals called endorphins.

In addition to the five senses, the brain also gets inputs from various parts of the internal body in order to regulate all of the functions that we are not normally conscious of, but which are necessary for staying alive.

BRAIN OUTPUTS

The brain outputs are bio-electrical signals which control internal bodily functions and the very large number of individual muscles which allow for motion, facial expressions, speech, and bodily functions basic to life. Speech is a particularly important function which involves output signals from the brain that operate the larynx, vocal cords, pharynx, soft palate, tongue, and lips, which are all necessary parts of the voice generation system. A feedback loop is established from the speech muscles and the ears to the brain that helps to achieve recognizable sounds and in learning how to speak. The vocal cords vibrate faster as they are pulled longer, thinner, and more taut, producing high frequency sound. They vibrate slower when they are shorter, thicker, and floppier, thereby producing lower frequency sounds. The pitch (frequency) range for the human voice is from about 60 HZto 2000HZ. Sound loudness has to do with the amount of air passing through the vocal cords.

The brain uses the central nervous system (CNS) for sending signals to and receiving information from the hundreds of muscles throughout the human body. The nerves of the CNS are actually axons of various lengths which propagate action potentials to muscles throughout the body. The CNS is the wiring harness of the human body. A typical muscle is made up of thousands of individual fibers and are controlled by what are called alpha motor neurons in either the brain or the spinal cord. A single alpha neuron can control hundreds of fibers as a unit. Special sensory stretch receptors called muscle spindles send information about the muscle state back to the brain thus creating a feedback loop resulting in smooth and controlled muscle response and movement. Some reflex movements take place between the spinal cord and the muscle, without the involvement of the brain. The portions of the brain involved with movement include the motor cortex, thalamus, basal ganglia, cerebrum, midbrain and brainstem. This gives us some idea of the importance of this function.

The nerve fiber (axon) terminates at a muscle fiber at a special structure called a neuromuscular junction, which is basically a synapse that connects the nerve fiber (electrical) to the muscle fiber (mechanical). An action potential propagating down the nerve releases the neurotransmitter, acetylcholine, which binds to receptors in the muscle fiber and stimulates the filaments (actin and myosin) in the muscle to slide across each other, thus shortening the muscle. Prior to stimulation the muscle is in a relaxed state. At the neuromuscular junction, the axon branches out into numerous terminal buttons that reside within depressions in what is called the motor end plate. It has been estimated that the spinal cord contains some 100 million neurons and their fibers.

It is amazing to realize that all of our human interactions and accomplishments have occurred by "merely" thinking, remembering, generating sounds, and moving body parts, as directed by the brain.

BRAIN PROCESSOR FUNCTIONS

The primary processing functions that the brain performs are sometimes described as MOVEMENT, EMOTION, MEMORY (LEARNING), LANGUAGE, AND SOCIALIZING. Another possible category might be THINKING which would include CREATIVITY. The information processor called the brain allows us to intelligently interact with our environment. It does this by means of sensory inputs which are then analyzed to formulate responses to those sensory inputs. However, the brain also has to process significant amounts of information from other internal sensors in order to maintain internal bodily functions basic to life. One example of this non-trivial activity is the gastro-intestinal tract. Eating is both a pleasurable and necessary activity, as we all know. The process of digestion is usually taken for granted, except when there are problems. Digestion involves some significant mechanical as well as complex chemical actions. Some scientists have estimated that the number of nerve cells involved in the gut, called the enteric nervous system, is far greater than previously believed. Communication between the brain and the gut occurs over the vagus nerve which contains a couple of thousand nerve fibers. We are reminded that the brain is involved with both internal and external functions when we "feel butterflies" in our stomachs, nervous stomachs, and various other stress related adverse effects on the digestive system.

Based on these relatively few but important abilities, the human species has come a long way. This chapter was an admittedly over-simplified, engineering oriented, look at the input/output and functional aspects of the brain. The purpose was to present the brain as an information processor, which it clearly is. By thinking of the brain as an information processor we can tend to de-mystify it and begin to make it more understandable to the average person.

Human Brain
Medial View

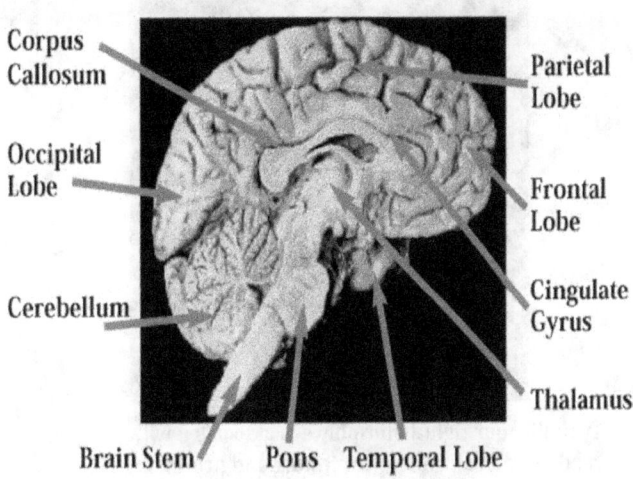

Corpus
Callosum

Occipital
Lobe

Cerebellum

Parietal
Lobe

Frontal
Lobe

Cingulate
Gyrus

Thalamus

Brain Stem   Pons   Temporal Lobe

Figure 3A

Where in the Brain?
Common Functions

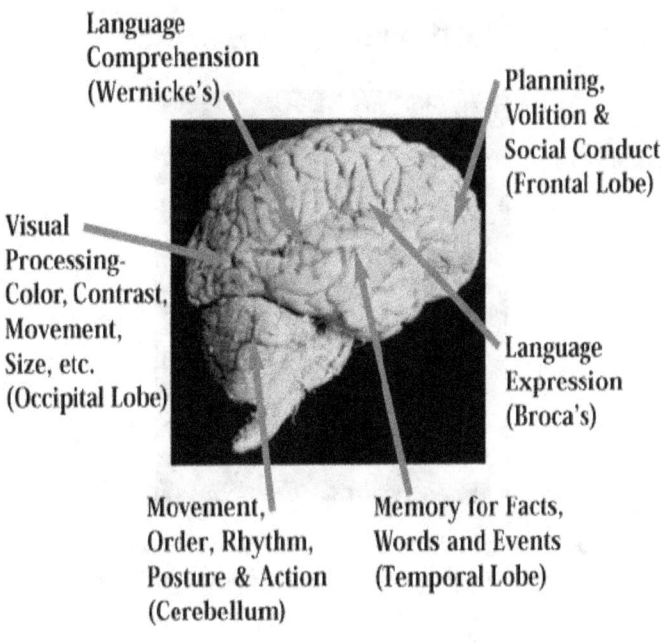

Language
Comprehension
(Wernicke's)

Visual
Processing-
Color, Contrast,
Movement,
Size, etc.
(Occipital Lobe)

Planning,
Volition &
Social Conduct
(Frontal Lobe)

Language
Expression
(Broca's)

Movement,
Order, Rhythm,
Posture & Action
(Cerebellum)

Memory for Facts,
Words and Events
(Temporal Lobe)

Figure 3B

Human Brain Functions
in the Right Hemisphere

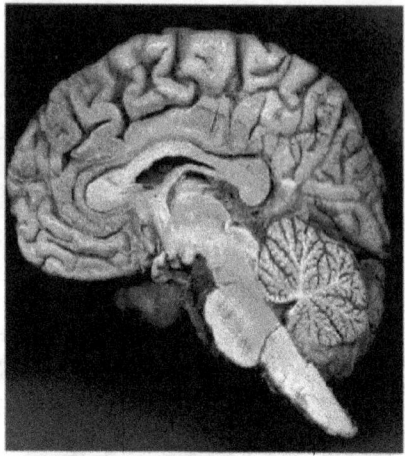

Typically, our right hemisphere is associated with
random, spatial, concrete thinking and processing of
"wholes". Contrary to popular belief, it is not necessarily
the creative hemisphere. In less than 5% of the population,
it processes language. More associated with "avoidance"
behaviors. Matures earlier in boys than it does in girls.

Figure 3C

Human Brain
Left Medial View

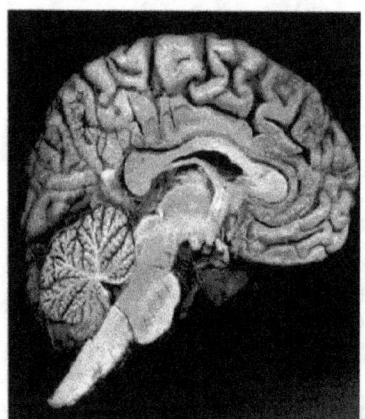

Typically, the left hemisphere of the brain is associated
with sequential and linear thinking. It processes "parts"
better than wholes. It is not innately logical. In over 95%
of the population, it processes language and "interprets"
our daily life. It matures earlier in girls than boys.

Figure 3D

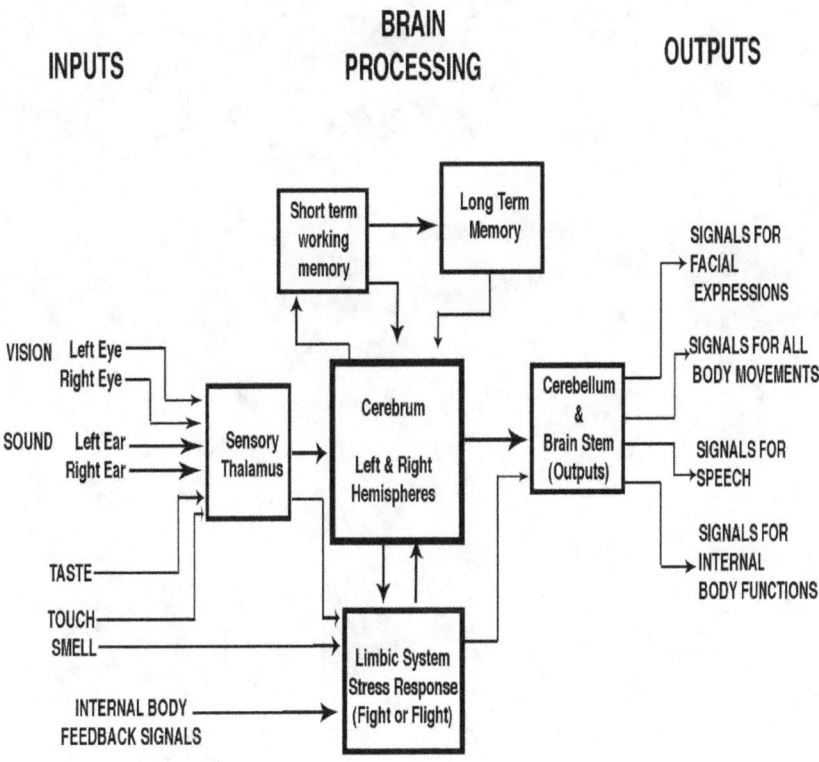

INPUTS

BRAIN PROCESSING

OUTPUTS

FIGURE 3E
BRAIN SIMPLIFIED BLOCK DIAGRAM

4

THE BIO-CHEMICAL BRAIN

The brain is a bio-chemical marvel, as is the rest of the human body. One of the most important chemical processes takes place in the synapses, which connect neurons and allow for one-way signal transmission. The chemicals that allow the synapses to function are called neurotransmitters. The chemical nature of neuronal transmission was suspected from studies dating back to the early 1900's. The first neurotransmitter to be discovered was acetylcholine in 1921 by a German biologist named Otto Loewi, who later won a Nobel prize for his work. Since that time over 50 neurotransmitters have been identified.

As far as signal processing characteristics are concerned, neurotransmitters come in two basic types. The excitatory types result in action potentials being generated in the post-synaptic neuron. The inhibitory type has the opposite effect, namely blocking or at least raising the effective threshold for the generation of an action potential. Inhibitory neurotransmitters are often called modulators since they have the ability to control activity in various areas of the brain. Neurons that activate inhibitory synapses are called inhibitory neurons as opposed to projection neurons which generate the action potentials which perform signal processing. Some neurotransmitters are synthesized in the cell body and transported in vesicles (containers) along the axon to the axon terminals, but most are synthesized at the axon terminals and stored there in synaptic vesicles. A neurotransmitter can have many functions.

The two neurotransmitters called glutamate (excitatory) and gaba (inhibitory), are responsible for most of the chemical signal processing in the brain. Other well-known modulator transmitters, called monoamines, include seratonin, dopamine, epinephrine, and norepinephrine. Unlike most other neurotransmitters, the cells which produce monoamines are found in only a few areas of the brain, mostly the brainstem, but the axons of these cells extend to widespread locations in the brain. These monoamines can thereby produce global state changes in multiple brain areas simultaneously, such as the high degree of arousal need in times of danger, or in the opposite direction as when we go to sleep. Acetylcholine is another monoamine which can function as either a fast transmitter or a modulator, with different post-synaptic receptors. Acetylcholine is a very important neurotransmitter in the body, involved with neurons that control muscle movements, including the heart muscles, and muscles in the gastro-intestinal tract.

The discoveries of specific neurotransmitters, and their specific roles in the functioning of the brain, ushered in a revolution in the way mental illness was to be treated. The medical term "chemical imbalance" has become commonplace for describing many brain disorders, and resulting drug treatments have continued to be introduced, with mixed results. The most well-known neurotransmitters considered most relevant to mental illnesses, and targeted by most of the drugs used in the treatment of brain disorders are dopamine and serotonin. The brain's main factory for dopamine are neurons in a tiny region of the brainstem called the substantia nigra, and these neurons project to many other areas of the brain. These are the neurons that are eventually destroyed in advanced Parkinson's disease. Dopamine is an inhibitory neurotransmitter and is involved in the attention and motivational systems, the reward system, and is thought to regulate emotional responses and play a role in schizophrenia and drug abuse. Schizophrenia and psychosis have been shown to involve excessive amounts of dopamine in the frontal lobes. On the other hand, too little dopamine in the motor areas of the brain are responsible for Parkinson's disease, which produces muscle tremors and progressively increasing problems with movements.

Seratonin is a modulator neurotransmitter believed to play many roles including temperature regulation, sensory perception, and the onset of sleep. It has also been found to be intimately involved in emotion and mood. Too little seratonin has been shown to lead to depression, problems with anger control, obsessive-compulsive disorder, and suicide. It is also believed that too little seratonin leads to an increased appetite for carbohydrates (starchy foods) and trouble sleeping, which are often associated with depression and other emotional disorders. A number of antidepressant drugs are targeted to brain seratonin systems and act to increase seratonin levels. Some antidepressant medications known as seratonin reuptake inhibitors work by blocking the reabsorption of seratonin by the pre-synaptic neuron, thus increasing the amount of seratonin available to the brain.

Depression is the most common of the so-called mood disorders. One class of drugs to treat depression are called monoamine inhibitors (MAOIs) and they increase the amount of norepinephrine available to receptors. Another drug type increases serotonin transmission and decreases acetylcholine transmission. A third group of drugs known as selective serotonin re-uptake inhibitors (SSRIs) which act to increase seratonin levels. As already discussed, seratonin is a modulator type of neurotransmitter widely used in the brain, and low levels of seratonin is associated with depression.

Another mood disorder called bipolar-disorder combines episodes of depression and hypomania (which can include psychosis). This disorder is usually treated with drugs that reduce dopamine transmission either by reducing dopamine release at the pre-synaptic terminal or by blocking receptors at the post-synaptic terminal. This same type of treatment is used for another very serious type of mental illness called schizophrenia. Parkinson's disease, a degenerative condition characterized by muscle rigidity and tremors is due to a loss of cells in the midbrain of the brainstem that produce and release dopamine. This is a classic case of too much or too little causing problems.

Norepinephrine, a modulator type neurotransmitter, is widely used in almost every region of the brain including the entire cortex, the hypothalamus, the cerebellum and the brain stem. Many of the medications used to treat mood disorders target the norepinephrine system

Neurotransmitters are the chemicals talked about in most discussions about the brain, but many less glamorous ones are also present in the brain performing important functions. Foremost among them is glucose (dextrose), a simple sugar that is the primary source of energy for the brain, and is supplied via the blood. Various salts including sodium, potassium, calcium and chloride are the electrically charged (ionic) particles that are basic to generating action potentials. These chemicals are found within the neuron cell membrane and in the cerebrospinal fluid (CSF) which is present throughout the brain and spinal cord. The CSF also helps to protect the brain from physical shock damage, and is contained within a membrane which surrounds the brain called the blood-brain barrier. This membrane also helps to filter out some unwanted chemicals from the many blood vessels which surround the brain.

Hormones are another class of chemicals that perform functions in both the brain and the rest of the body. Hormones are made of protein produced and released by various glands, and they circulate in the bloodstream in order to reach their target cells, which they stimulate in various ways. Certain hormones have functions in the brain and are called neurohormones. In the chapter 6 on stress we will talk about the pituitary gland which is physically very close to the hypothalamus in the brain and which produces the hormone that initiates the stress (fight-or-flight) response. Another hormone is fed-back to the brain to provide the signal for turning off the stress-response. Neurotransmitters and hormones are therefore very similar classes of chemicals, with the main difference being that the neurotransmitters work in the neuron synapses and the hormones work in the bloodstream, which in some ways could be considered one very large synapse.

A lot of chemical processes take place within the neuron's cell body, under the direction of DNA within the cell. The cell is a mini chemical factory. Biology and chemistry are obviously two of the important scientific fields basic to brain research. But as we will discuss in the next chapter, a significant part of the brain's processing is bio-electrical.

The field of biological psychiatry has grown out of the assumption that mental disorders are due to chemical imbalances in the brain. This is a theory which is hard to dispute based on the known degree to which brain functioning is based on bio-chemical means, but it is certainly an over-simplified explanation of mental illness. Because of limited diagnostic ability, as well as inability to limit the drug action to specific brain areas, this process is a trial-and-error one with serious side effects not being uncommon. With both psychiatrists and other medical doctors commonly prescribing these drugs, their use has exploded and new drugs are continuously being introduced. It is very unfortunate that profit motives are putting far more emphasis on finding new drugs rather than on basic brain research. Until we know more about how the brain works, the optimal treatments, or better yet, the means for prevention of brain disorders will not be found.

The topic of drugs is an important one in any discussion of the brain. The word drug has undergone an interesting evolution even within my lifetime. In the 1950's the word drug was respectable and every neighborhood had its pharmacy, usually referred to as the drug store. In those days, however, the volume of drug sales, both prescription and over-the-counter were far less than today, because fewer were available and fewer visits to the doctor were made. In the 1970's with the increase in illegal drug use, the word "drug" took on a mostly negative connotation. Justifiably, a "war on drugs" was launched, but it would become another one of the un-winnable wars. Then gradually came the new drug revolution, this one by the traditional medical community, bolstered by the pharmaceutical companies. It almost seems like the plan was to flood the market with legal drugs as a way to eliminate the competition from illegal drugs. This certainly happened with the drug called alcohol. There is little or no illegal competition to the alcoholic beverage industry. So today the word drug recovers its positive meaning, and our government even passes a medicare drug benefit plan to make more drugs available to more people. We are clearly in the miracle-drug mode, consistent with the quick-fix mentality for problem-solving, which is more often good for profits and not patients. The only logical, albeit long-term solution to these problems is goal-oriented neuroscience research.

The predominantly chemical nature of the brain and the ability of certain substances to change the way we feel and behave has been known for ages. Until more recently, however, these substances were derived from natural and limited sources, primarily from plants or as in the case of alcohol, from relatively simple processes. With the advancement of technology and the dramatic growth of the pharmaceutical industry, the situation has changed dramatically. Now an almost unlimited variety of chemicals can be formulated, and new markets for drugs are constantly being explored. For example, there is now a new fancy name for a class of drugs called cognitive enhancement drugs. For example, if someone believes he or she can get a competitive advantage by improving their attention span, or by reducing their anxiety in meeting new people, they could ask a doctor to prescribe a drug which previously was intended for treatment of disorders. A similar situation is going on in baseball, and other sports, with performance enhancement substances such as steroids, for example. This is all somewhat uncharted territory and carry both health and even ethical implications. The situation borders on being out of control. The fact is that the full scope of the long-term effects of drugs are not always uncovered in clinical trials. There is no substitute for a sound scientific understanding of exactly how a new drug works in the brain and the rest of the body, before approval, but this rarely happens. The physician's desk reference (the bible of information about approved drugs) is loaded with descriptions of drugs with the statement that the exact mechanism by which the drug works is "unknown".

Our bio-chemical brains are amazingly robust as a result of impressive design characteristics, but unfortunately it is at the same time subject to damage by both physical and chemical threats. The brain needs the optimum amount of exercise and good nutrition just as the rest of the body does. A working knowledge of neuroscience is not beyond the reach of the average person, and keeping up with scientific advances will help us to keep our brains as healthy as possible.

5

THE BIO-ELECTRICAL BRAIN

We know that information transmission and processing in the brain has both electrical and chemical components. The electro/chemical characteristics of the brain began to be discussed over 200 years ago, but it wasn't until 1952 that A.L. Hodgkin and A. Huxley published a paper in which they presented the first intercellular recording of the neuron's impulse (action potential) in the giant squid axon. They also presented a mathematical model for calculation of nerve impulse generation. Mathematical modeling of the neuron's bio-electrical properties is complex because of the highly non-linear properties of the neuron. This was the beginning of the modern field of membrane biophysics.

The component part of the brain's circuitry that most clearly exhibits the integration of both chemical and electrical processes is the synapse, which was introduced in chapter 2. Some purely electrical synapses appear in the brain, but most are of the chemical variety. A very simplified drawing of how the chemical synapse produces an electrical output is shown in figure 5a. When neurotransmitters are released into the synaptic space, some of them bind to receptors on the post-synaptic membrane. The

receptors are highly specific to chemical inputs. When a receptor receives a chemical input a channel is opened through the membrane which allows charged molecules, called ions, to enter the dendrite which initiates a process resulting in a "spike" of ionic current and the generation of what is called an "excitatory post-synaptic potential" (EPSP), or sometimes called a "generator potential". The process of generating an EPSP at the post-synaptic terminal is similar to the process that occurs in the neuron, at what is called the "trigger zone" where the cell body transitions to the axon terminal, producing a similar but larger ionic burst called an "action potential".

We now know a lot about the action potential produced by neurons and which propagates along the neuron's axon to the multiple synaptic terminals at the ends of the axon branches. It is the fundamental electrical signal used in all of the brain's circuitry. The waveform of the action potential is shown in figure 5b. It has a peak amplitude of about 110 millivolts and a pulse width of about 1 millisecond. The neuron acts as a threshold device in that it produces the action potential when the combined inputs from the dendrites causes the cell body potential to increase above a threshold excitation level. This process is illustrated in figure 5c, starting with the synapses. The generator potentials produced at the synapse outputs are much smaller versions of the action potential and are only a few millivolts in amplitude. It takes multiple generator potentials occurring simultaneously to trigger an action potential. There is about a 0.5-1 millisecond signal transmission delay through the chemical synapse, and it takes about 1 millisecond for a synapse to clear of neurotransmitters and be ready for a next impulse.

The generator potentials are in effect added together (summation) in the post-synaptic cell until a threshold level is exceeded at the trigger zone between the cell body and the axon, at which time an action potential is generated and propagates down the axon. There is about a 1-3 millisecond period after an action potential before another pulse can be generated, due to the reset characteristics of the voltage-gated ion channels. This, together with the approximately 1 millisecond width on the action potential, limits the maximum firing rate of action potentials to about 100 per second (100 HZ). However, a frequency modulation range of 1 to 100 HZ still represents a significant information coding capability.

We need to remember that synapses can be either excitatory or inhibitory, depending on the neurotransmitter involved, meaning that they either encourage or discourage the generation of an action potential in the post-synaptic neuron. Excitatory post-synaptic gates usually involve sodium inflow whereas inhibitory gates usually involve potassium or chloride outflow. Inhibitory actions can last from milliseconds to seconds.

Each neuron is a mini information processor, in that it accepts inputs and generates an output. The inputs come via the neuron's dendrites and their synaptic connections to preceding neurons. The output is delivered via the neuron's axon and synaptic connections to other following neurons. The neuron cell body has the ability to generate an electrical impulse (action potential) which is analogous to the 1 or 0 (on/off) action of binary coding and logic circuitry in electronics signal processing. In the "OFF" state the voltage inside a neuron is about -65mv relative to the outside of the cell membrane. As it receives dendrite inputs (in the form of charged ions) the inside voltage rises (becomes more positive). When it reaches a voltage of about -40mv a process starts that generates an electrical impulse that travels down the axon at the relatively slow rate of about 200 feet per second, since it is an electro-chemical as opposed to electrical only transmission, as in a conductor (wire) which happens at the speed of light. Most axons are relatively short, therefore transmission delay through them is basically negligible. The electrical phenomena occurring in living things is usually called BIOELECTRICITY.

The action potential of the neuron is generated by charged atoms (ions), and in particular positively charged sodium and potassium ions. An ion is an electrically charged element which migrates freely in solution, and is responsible for the electrical conductivity of the solution. Negative charges for the axon's inactive state are derived from chloride ions. It is the "pumping" of these ions across cell membranes which results in voltage changes. The electrical impulse (action potential) generated is of fixed amplitude. Information is contained in the absence or presence of a pulse, as well as in the frequency (or rate) of firing. In electrical engineering terminology, the neuron provides a "thresholding" and "switching" characteristic which is similar to logic and other signal processing circuitry in man-made electronics systems.

Scientists are working to understand more about the neuron's dendrites and dendrite spines which are microscopic outgrowths which connect the input synapses to the dendrite branch and thereby to the neuron cell body. Spines are present in large numbers in most neurons and they receive most excitatory inputs thus mediating the transfer of synaptic potentials to the dendrite shaft and then to the cell body for integration with the other dendrite signals. Researchers have speculated that dendrite spines play a key electrical role in the transmission of synaptic potentials (EPSPs or generator potentials). It has been proposed that spines might systematically alter synaptic inputs either by amplifying or filtering EPSPs, or by serving as low-pass filters. It is clear to researchers that spines are more than passive compartments. An abundance of recent data hints at the rich diversity of ion channels that exist on the spine head, yet the exact electrical function for spines is still unknown. As is the overall brain, the tiny dendrite spine is apparently itself some combination of chemical and electrical.

Using only the basic circuit elements discussed above, the brain might seem like a relatively uncomplicated device. But the interconnections into circuits and networks become very complex, with billions of neurons involved. This basic concept of simple circuit elements connected into various configurations has some similarities to the digital computer, but with processing speeds much slower than computers. However, the brain appears to use many individual processors working in parallel, which increases its overall processing capabilities.. A field or research dating back to the 1950s, called neural networks, has been investigating how neurons might be connected to perform signal processing functions. Neural networks are quantitative models linking inputs and outputs adaptively in a learning process that is believed to simulate what happens in the human brain. These networks have been shown to perform many brain type signal processing functions, such as facial recognition and many others. Work is on-going in this field led by cognitive psychologists, statisticians, engineers, and mathematicians. Unfortunately, neural networks are so different from the binary/digital circuitry of computers, that the research tends not to attract much attention. One has to wonder why there seems to be no significant applications for man-make neural network type information processors.

A brain circuit is a group of neurons linked together by synaptic connections. A network is a group of circuits that together perform a particular brain function. Some researchers have speculated that the neurons are in a constant state of random firing (noise) and are turned on by any electrical activity around them such as the firing of nearby but unconnected neurons. This situation changes when a real signal comes along, at which time the neurons fire much more rapidly and in synchronized ways. By this description our brains are always filled with noise-like activity until real sensory inputs arrive and predominate above the noise. This may be true to some degree, but we know from recent "PET" scan data that one can clearly recognize the difference between in-active and active portions of the brain. As an engineer, this means to me that there is a good amount of noise immunity in the signal processor called the brain.

Scientists have known for a long time that the brain has an electrical component to its functioning, as evidenced by "shock treatment", technically known as electro convulsive therapy, or ECT, which has been around since the 1930s and is still in use today, although controversial. ECT often produces memory disturbances as a side-effect. A related treatment, called rapid transcranial magnetic stimulation or RTMS, creates a current in the brain by using a magnetic field that crosses the exterior of the skull. Other more invasive electrical treatments used in rare cases, called deep brain stimulation, involve electrodes implanted directly into a particular part of the brain. Today's electrical or chemical treatments of brain disorders are not as effective as we would want, primarily because of our limited understanding of how the brain works. It is reasonable to expect that when more is known about the brain, and medical technology advances to provide easier access to all parts of the brain, new ways of treating most brain disorders will emerge. It is clear to me that we need more engineers (especially electrical) involved in brain research in order to accelerate progress.

Interestingly, besides chemical and electrical processes, the brain also has some very important "mechanical" features. This mechanical aspect shows up in the various forms of "gates" (also called channels) which are basically valves that turn on or off the flow of chemicals, namely neurotransmitters or ionic elements. These gates are controlled by chemical receptors, as in synapses and dendrites, or by voltage levels as in the axon membrane, where action potentials are generated. These very important "mini-components of the brain are analogous to their all electrical counterparts in electronics design called the field-effect transistor (FET), which is also used for on/off gating functions. The brain's mechanical gates are much slower speed than the FET, but obviously adequate for the overall relatively slow-speed operation of the brain, which we now have to call the chemical/electrical/mechanical central processing unit of the human body.

FIGURE 5 (a) SYNAPSE CHEMICAL TO ELECTRICAL CONVERSION

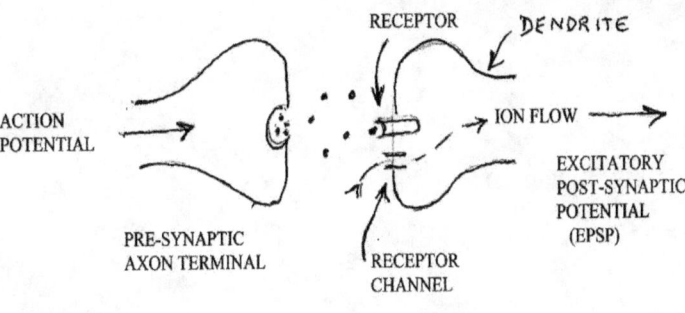

FIGURE 5 (b)   NEURON ACTION POTENTIAL

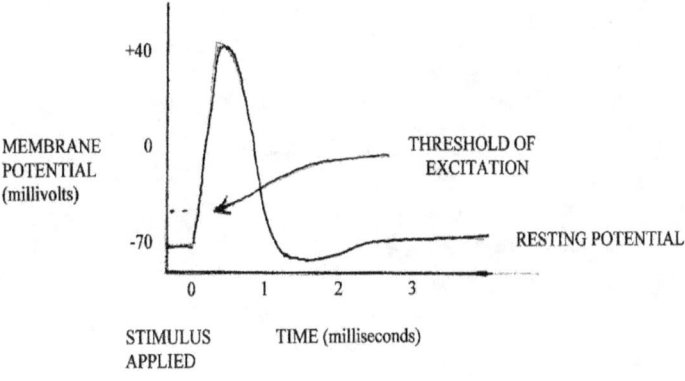

FIGURE 5 (c)   NEURON'S SIGNAL FLOW

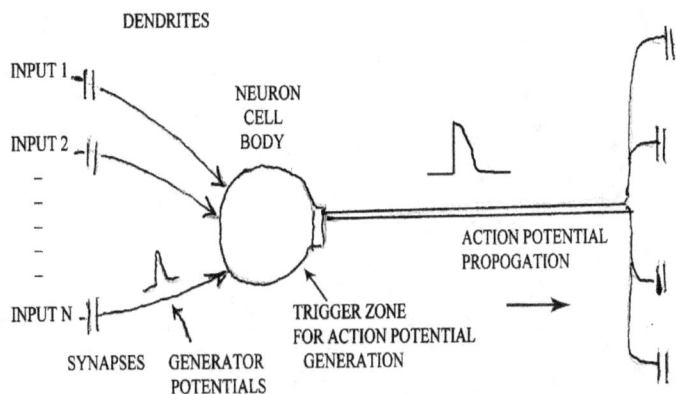

6

THE STRESS RESPONSE
AND EMOTIONS

Staying alive is a high priority for all organisms, therefore having a brain function for rapidly sensing danger and then taking action is highly desirable. However, the nature of threats has changed significantly since the cave-man days, but our brain and body mechanisms for reacting to them has not changed. This mismatch between modern society and our brains is believed to be a major contributor to mental illness today.

The system that we have for detecting and responding to danger is commonly called the LIMBIC SYSTEM which produces the well-known "fight-or-flight" response, more recently known as the "stress response", which is more descriptive of its present day application. The central portion of the brain (which is referred to as the EMOTIONAL CENTER in the last chapter) is where our emotional circuitry is located, with the two most important structures involved being the AMYGDALA and HIPPOCAMPUS.

A frightening experience activates the amygdala immediately, even before it is analyzed by the thinking part of the brain (the cortex). The amygdala signals the hypothalamus which releases a chemical which activates the body's hormonal system designed to prepare the body for action. The two glands involved in this system are the pituitary, located just below the hypothalamus, and the adrenal glands, which are located near the kidneys. It is the adrenal glands which release adrenaline (also called epinephrine), which increases heart and breathing rates, and also release steroids such as cortisol, which helps keep up blood sugar, giving the body extra energy to act. Working with the amygdala, the hippocampus forms memories of these emotional events. A negative feedback loop exists back to the brain in order to shut down the stress response and restore balance in the body when the threat has passed. A block diagram of this important integrated brain/body function is shown in figure 6.

The bad news from research scientists is that chronic (prolonged) stress, with its over-activation of the stress response, can damage both the brain and the body. Stress can contribute to heart disease and digestive diseases, and weaken the immune system. Stress can be a trigger, if not a direct cause of many mental illnesses. Recent research has shown that stress and the resulting excessive release of cortisol can damage the hippocampus. To make matters even worse, unhealthy coping mechanisms such as smoking, excessive alcohol, and illegal drugs can multiply the damaging effects of stress. Some psychologists have defined four coping levels to asses one's stress status. They are as follows;

1. Stressed Out / Burned Out

Severe difficulties in coping, incapacitating feelings of anxiety, dread, depression, helplessness and/or anger, impaired functioning on the job or in personal life, extreme distress, presence of physical symptoms such as sleep and/or appetite disturbance, lowered immunity, physical tension, or depleted energy.

2. Strained

Frequent difficulty in coping, a sense of overwhelm or feeling drained, persistent feelings of anxiety, anger, irritability, helplessness, worry, gloom, some impairment in functioning at work or personal life.

3. Balanced

Effective and relatively stable functioning at work and/or personal life. Occasional distressing feelings which are appropriate and minimally disturbing or disruptive.

4. Highly Effective

Highly effective and creative problem solving and performancel, feeling challenged, energized, motivated, anticipating successful resolution.

Most of us would probably say that we have been in each of these modes at one time or another, and strive for more time in level 4. An important question to ask is how much stress can one take without adverse health effects. This is where the issues of stressors and stress-resistance become important. It is logical to assume that the two main contributors to one's degree of stress resistance are 1) our general state of physical health, and 2) our personality traits. The title of this chapter is "Stress and Emotions". It could have been called "Stress and Personality", since our personalities are defined by how we feel and express our emotions and how we react to situations. The real issue then, in terms of tolerable stress level, is the difference between the level of stress we are under, which we can call "total stress", compared to our "stress tolerance level". Determining our stress tolerance level would require some kind of comprehensive personality evaluation test. Then the next logical question for most of us to ask is how we can increase our stress tolerance level. If it comes down to needing to change some personality trait, the good news is that it may be possible, but will take hard work. Fortunately, the brain is re-programmable to a large degree.

The strong message is to learn how to keep stress under control. Certainly this is easier said than done. For those of us who have stress-prone personalities, the changes are not easy to bring about, but if achieved they can be life-saving. Finding relaxation techniques that work for us can be very helpful. Many different forms of relaxation are available, and they are all able to initiate what is called the "relaxation response" which can be considered a way to turn-down the stress-response, temporarily at least. Another positive input from the most recent brain research is that the brain has a great deal of "plasticity" which is the ability to change itself by growing neurons and by re-wiring brain circuitry. This means that with motivation, concentration and effort we can replace unhealthy stress responses with healthy ones. Our personalities are apparently not cast in concrete, which means that anyone may be able to learn how to develop more stress-resistant personality traits.

The brain and the rest of the human body clearly were designed to handle some amount of stress, as indicated by the extent of the stress response system. This system is a good example of how the brain and the rest of the body work as one unit to accomplish a task that is fundamental to our survival. But the chronic stress conditions associated with modern-day society can go beyond our capabilities to adapt. Both chronic and acute stress can be a trigger, if not the basic cause of many mental illnesses. It seems to me that learning how to develop stress-resistant personalities needs to be part of our educational system. This would have to start at the earliest possible age, since the evidence is that our personalities are established early in life. Once established, personalities are not easy to change. Psychologists have identified certain characteristics of people who achieve positive health, and would clearly be stress-resistant to a high degree. These characteristics include;

1) self acceptance

2) positive relations with others

3) autonomy, or the ability to regulate one's life according to personal standards and not the opinions and approval of others

4) the ability to choose and create environments that are conducive to happiness

5) having a purpose in life

6) a strong sense of personal growth

We all know that a healthy diet, adequate exercise, and a good night's sleep are also basic ingredients to stress-reduction and good health in general. But knowing is one thing, doing is considerably harder. The stress response system is a good example of how integrated the brain is with the rest of the body. Interactions between the brain and the rest of the body are constantly going on, however, it is the brain alone which generates our emotions and makes the lifestyle decisions that are often unhealthy. As mentioned before, personality and behavior are closely related, and one could think of personality as the most important brain software program, that we start installing early in life. We still don't know how much of our personalities are genetic and how much is learned (environmental). We do know that personality traits are difficult to change, but not necessarily impossible, if the motivation is strong enough.

Emotions originate in the brain and can be kept there or expressed in various ways. Certain emotions can result in actions which are harmful to ourselves and others. The range of human emotions are often considered to include four basic ones, namely fear, anger, sadness and joy. Other emotions are considered from combinations of these four. For example, worry, anxiety and stress all derive mostly from fear, with a little anger and/or sadness thrown in. It is easy to conclude that any of these emotions can range from healthy to unhealthy depending on the degree and time duration as well as the way they are expressed. For example, although anger is a normal emotion, it can become a problem if felt too intensely or frequently, or if expressed inappropriately in some overly aggressive way.

An excellent reference for a much more detailed discussion of human emotions is the book by Joseph LeDoux called "The Emotional Brain". He points out that both nature and nurture contribute to our emotional make-up, and that emotions, especially fear, had very important survival value early in our evolution. Unfortunately we now have more fears than we need, and they account for many common psychiatric problems today, including anxiety disorders, obsessive-compulsive disorder, post-traumatic stress disorder, and various phobias. Emotions are universal, and bodily expressions (especially of the face) occurring during emotions are similar for people around the world. Professor LeDoux points out that the human brain is the product of evolutionary tinkering, and that presently the pathways from the amygdala to the cortex overshadow the pathways from the cortex to the amygdala. He speculates that with future evolutionary increases in connectivity between the cortex and amygdala, cognition and emotion might begin to work together rather than separately, giving a more harmonious integration of reason and passion. But meanwhile, as we learn more about how the brain works and about brain plasticity, we can hopefully do a better job of programming our brains for improved performance.

Thinking of the brain as an information processor with inputs and outputs, we realize that emotions are the responses (outputs) to emotional stimuli (inputs). From this information systems perspective, if there are problems with this overall system, the logical thing to do is modify the processor. Fortunately, the brain has some degree of re-programmability (plasticity) as will be discussed in chapter 7. As neuroscientists learn more about the brain and plasticity, we may develop more effective ways of re-programming our brains for more stress-resistant personalities.

FIGURE 6 STRESS RESPONSE

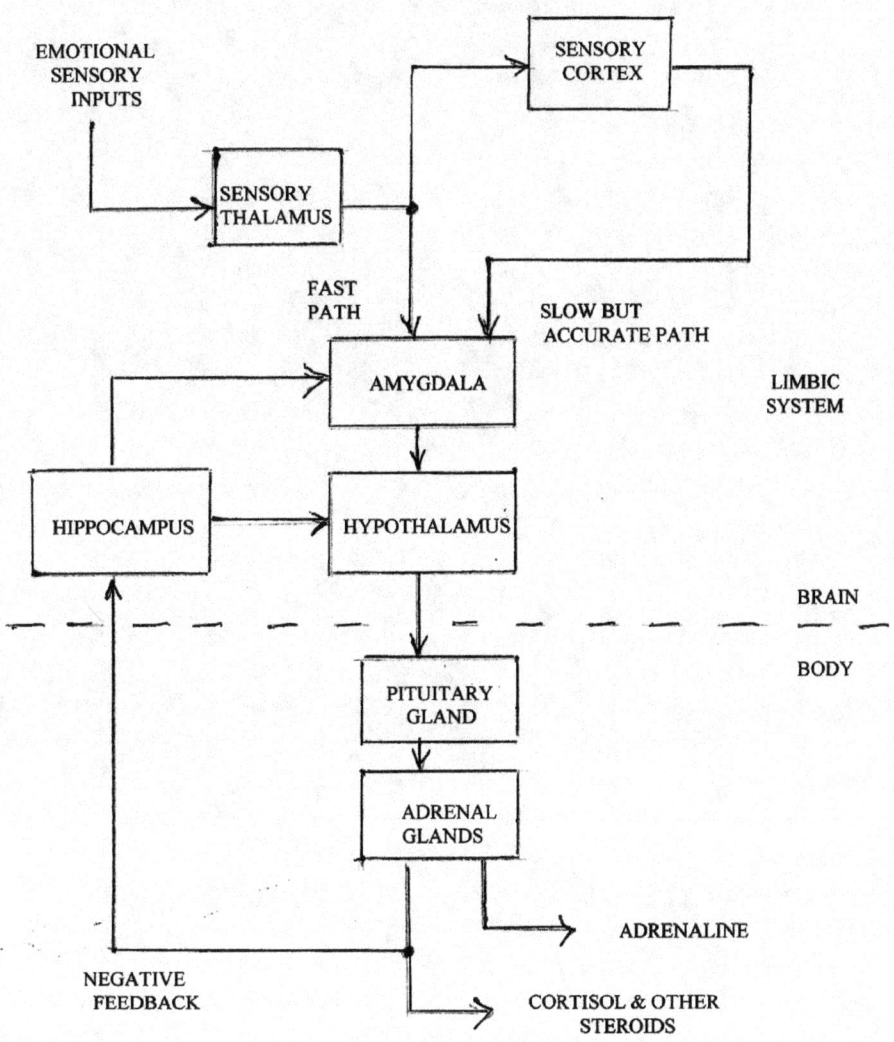

7

PLASTICITY
AND PROGRAMMING

Neuroplasticity (or brain plasticity) refers to the ability of neurons to make new connections, which in effect means re-wiring of the brain. It also means the ability of the brain to produce new neurons. Scientists now believe that even the adult brain can do both of these things. Clearly genetics plays a role in how the brain is wired, but environmental factors (experience) are also important. Learning is a brain re- configuration process. The hardware of the brain appears to be dynamic and malleable throughout life, with the ability to both learn and un-learn. In a sense, both learning and memory are examples of brain plasticity, and in computer jargon could be equated to programming.

Some neuroscientists define plasticity, or neuroplasticity, as the lifelong ability of the brain to reorganize neural pathways based on new experiences. Another way to think of plasticity is the ability of the brain to change with learning. Plasticity has an age dependent determinant, and can also compensate for lost function and/or maximize remaining function in the event of brain injury. Neuroscientists estimate that at birth each neuron in the cerebral cortex has approximately 2,500 synapses, and that the number grows to about 15,000 at about age three years old. This is about twice the amount in the adult brain. As we age, old connections are deleted through a process called "synaptic pruning". Experience determines which connections will be strengthened and which will be pruned. Connections which are activated most frequently will be preserved.

The Canadian psychologist, Donald Hebb, in his 1949 book, "The Organization of Behavior", is credited with first proposing the synaptic theory of memory, and which is now called "Hebbian plasticity". His proposal was that "when an axon of cell A is near enough to excite cell B, or repeatedly and consistently takes part in firing it, some growth process or metabolic changes take place in one or both cells such that A's efficiency, as one of the cells firing B, is increased". In 1973 a paper was published which described the phenomenon of long-lasting potentiation, now called long-term potentiation (LTP), in which actual experiments were described in which a stimulating electrode was put in the fiber pathway going into the hippocampus, and a recording electrode in the hippocampus itself. It was found that following the potentiating pulses, the synaptic response got bigger relative to the baseline response, and remained bigger for hours. In recent years thousands of papers have been published on this topic, however, the specifics of how memory really works is still unknown.

The fact that even adults are able to learn, and that learning reflects changes in the brain, indicates that the brain retains some of its plasticity throughout life. We now know that the adult brain also has some ability to grow new neurons and to do some amount of repair of damaged areas. The neurons that pack our brain at birth continue to connect themselves into circuits throughout our lives. By using the power of attention, we can slowly rewire our brain circuitry, and both learn and unlearn. This gives us great power for change.

A very readable book on the subject of plasticity is "The Mind and the Brain, Neuroplasticity and the Power of Mental Force", by Jeffrey M. Schwartz, M.D., and Sharon Begley. Although Dr. Schwartz's research is primarily aimed at obsessive compulsive disorder (OCD), the implications are much broader and may apply to many other mental illnesses as well. If the brain can be re-wired (re-programmed), then we can replace damaging thought processes with healthy ones. This process takes hard work which Dr. Schwartz calls mental force, but the result can be a real and permanent cure, as opposed to the temporary symptom relief and usually non-insignificant side-effects of most drug treatments. This non-drug type of treatment is called behavioral, or cognitive therapy, and has none of the adverse side-effect problems of drug therapies.

One of the most important programs that we install in our brains primarily during childhood, is the one called personality. It is our personality that largely determines how we react to our environment, and we have already discussed the significant advantages of having a stress-resistant personality. Some experts believe that one's basic personality traits are unchangeable, but it is still debatable as to how much one can change his or her personality later in life. The concept of plasticity gives us hope that change is possible, if the motivation to change is strong enough. The medical profession, in my opinion, is avoiding the personality issue by relying on the less controversial chemical imbalance explanation for disorders, without explaining what causes the chemical imbalance in the first place. A prescription for a drug and a follow-up appointment may be the norm for present day treatments, but it is both risky and inadequate.

Brain plasticity is one of the truly astounding characteristics of the brain, and it has allowed the same basic design to adapt to millions of years of changes in the lives of humans. Experiences effect the brain when they are stored as synaptic changes, and possibly other changes, in one or more systems of the brain during learning, which is why research on synaptic plasticity, and on learning and memory, is so important. Efficient utilization of the large cortex of the human species has allowed dramatic advancements. The development of a complex language is probably the single most important factor in the optimum utilization of this brain power, and the resulting overall positive effect on the species. Unfortunately, different groups of humans developed different languages, whereas one universal language would have been the optimum. The other basic advantage of the human brain compared to all the rest is the immense capacity for memory storage. Memory is not only a basic requirement for human consciousness, it is also a necessary ability for learning and creativity. As important as memory is, however, we still do not know much about how memory really works, or what the memory capacity of the human brain might be. As scientists learn more about how the brain works, we will hopefully learn more about how brain plasticity might be enhanced. This will be applicable in the field of education and might be one of the most important benefits of increased investments in brain research. We are already seeing a lot of information becoming available under the name of "brain-based learning". The potential is very significant and this alone justifies an increase in priority and funding for neuroscience research.

8

GENETICS PLUS ENVIRONMENT

The brain that we wind up with as adults is a product of both genetics (inheritance) and environment (diet, lifestyle, education, etc.). Unfortunately, science cannot as yet tell us exactly how much each factor contributes to the process. There may come a time in the foreseeable future when genetic testing will be able to accurately predict predispositions to, and our risk of developing various mental illnesses. This would allow possible preventative measures to be taken which would prevent the illness from developing. At some time in the future there may also be effective methods for modifying genes and even replacing defective genes. The best of genes, however, is not a guarantee of protecting us from environmental risk factors.

Genetics is the scientific discipline that studies heredity and searches for the basic principles governing inheritance. Genetic scientists have had to work their way down to the cellular level to unlock some of the secrets of heredity. A basic principle of biology is that all organisms are either single cells or complexes of cells, and that a cell is a basic biological unit, a structure bounded by a membrane that separates the cell interior from the outside environment. The cell is considered to be the basic unit of life, and living things may be defined as things that are made up of cells. The human body is made up of as least 100 different types of cells, and is estimated to have a total of about 100 trillion cells. Each type of cell is responsible for a specific task.

Inside every cell of our bodies (except red blood cells) is a relatively dense structure called the nucleus. The nucleus is especially important because it contains the chromosomes, which are the structures that contain the stuff of heredity, namely our genes. Genes reside on chromosomes and are made of DNA (deoxyribonucleic acid). Human cells contain 46 chromosomes (23 pairs), in the well-known double-helix shape, and comprising what is commonly called the DNA molecule. We inherit half of our chromosomes from each parent. The genetic code refers to the 100,000 or so genes located on the 23 pairs of chromosomes. Every cell in each human body contains the same DNA and the same genes. The codes stored in DNA are in effect a database. The double strands of DNA can separate and act as templates for two fundamental purposes. The first function of DNA is duplication of the entire pair of strands in the double helix, in order to transfer the complete database to new offspring cells. The second major function of DNA is for production of proteins and other chemicals needed by the cells to perform their overall functions. RNA is a copy of the DNA and is made in the cell nucleus and travels to the cytoplasm section of the cell where proteins are made. DNA is composed of only four chemical bases, called nucleotides, and labeled A, C, G, and T (for adenine, cytosine, guamine, and thiamine). These four bases are the biochemical embodiment of our genes.

The genetic code is estimated to have about 100,000 genes, but there are estimated to be 100,000,000,000 (one hundred billion) neurons, with as many as 1,000,000,000,000 (one trillion) connections between them. The brain is able to be represented by its relatively small number of genes because there are general patterns of design that are repeatedly used throughout the brain, thus reducing the amount of information required for their specification and generation.

Genes are instructional manuals or blueprints for our bodies. The human genome is the structure of the DNA and all the genes within it, and contains instructions for body development as well as the development of the overall structure of the brain. It is believed that 70% of all genes in the human body are related to brain cell activity. The genes control the manufacture within our cells of the basic substances that make up the human body, namely proteins, enzymes, nucleic acids and thousands of biochemicals. Proteins are the machines that make all living things function. Each cell may contain thousands of different proteins, which are long chains of twenty or so basic molecules known as amino acids, which consist of combinations of carbon, hydrogen, oxygen and nitrogen atoms. The process whereby genes "turn-on" to exert their influence on the cell is called gene expression, and it is believed to be controlled by a combination of in-born as well as environmental factors. Expressed genes are first translated into messenger RNA (ribonucleic acid) and then translated into proteins. An average cell has thousands of different proteins which are molecules that are necessary for the structure, function and regulation of the body's cells. Proteins may function as hormones, enzymes, and antibodies. Proteomics is the scientific study of all the proteins produced by genomes.

Genes play an important role throughout life with respect to controlling cellular activity, but experience can apparently modify gene expression. It is safe to say that the overall pattern of brain development is under both genetic and environmental (non-genetic) control. It is believed that genes contribute at most 50% to a given trait and in many instances probably far less. Learning is a process by which experience modifies the brain by modifying the expression of genes. The field of study on how genes express themselves to result in a biological function is called "functional genomics". The overall field of genetics (including genetic engineering) is rapidly expanding and provides an exciting career choice for science-oriented students, who have an interest in biology and chemistry.

Certain diseases have been linked to genetic factors, and genes can predispose people in certain directions without predetermining an outcome. Much effort is underway to determine exactly the extent to which genes contribute to mental illness. Genetics will continue to be an important field of medical research for helping to find cures and means of preventing many diseases. But we also need to continue to study the effects of environment on health, including diet and lifestyle. Humans need to take in nutrients in order to maintain life. We were designed with elaborate digestive systems that are able to extract the nutrients that are needed for maintaining life. Diet requirements for optimum health are hotly debated between the traditional and alternative medical communities. Food allergies obviously need to be taken into account, as well as personal tastes. America's free enterprise system has created the modern supermarket, which can be described as a minefield of attractively packaged but downright dangerous foods.

One of the most important environmental factors in our lives is education, which has a major impact on the development of the brain. One can think of education (learning) as brain programming. Brains vary significantly in their learning abilities, and a variety of factors contribute to our particular educational interests. The societies that work the best provide a wide variety of career opportunities for their citizens. As we learn more about how the brain works and how it develops, both parents and teachers will be able to do a better job in preparing children for productive, satisfying, and healthy adult lives.

9

BRAIN MONITORING
AND IMAGING

The first practical instrument designed to monitor and analyze brain activity was the electroencephalo-gram (EEG) which dates back to the early 1900s. This device was based on the fact that the tissues of the body conduct electricity, and that metal sensors placed on the skin could pick up the electrical activity of the brain, and these signals could be amplified and printed out or displayed on a monitor. With the EEG, four types of brain waves were found to exist in normal people called alpha, beta, theta, and delta waves. The frequency range and brain state associated with EEG brain waves are as follows:

	Frequency Range (hz)	State of Brain
DELTA	0.5 - 4	Deep Sleep
THETA	4 - 8	Drowsiness
ALPHA	8 - 14	Relaxed but Alert
BETA	14 - 30	Highly Alert and Focused

Another technique for monitoring brain waves is called Magnetoencephalography (MEG), and uses sensors on the skull to detect magnetic fields generated by electrical activity in activated neurons. Both EEG and MEG technologies can differentiate between certain gross states of consciousness, but have very limited value for diagnosing brain disorders. They have been complemented in recent years by the newer types of neuroimaging technologies, with the first being the X-ray machine, which evolved into the CAT (computerized-axial-topography) scanner, or simply the CT (computed topography) scanner in the 1970s. CT is based on the "blunting" or attenuation effect of the x-rays being a function of tissue density. CT scanners contain powerful computers for processing the information and creating the images. Recently, I had to have a CT scan of my brain and two "slices" of the scans are shown at the end of this chapter. They are useful to radiologists and neurologists for detecting certain abnormalities. I was told that my scans were considered "normal" for my age group.

The next significant development in brain imaging took place in the 1980s with magnetic resonance imaging (MRI). Using electro-magnetism rather that X-rays, the MRI is better for soft-tissue imaging, and has very high resolution. MRI is based on the fact that the protons of cells when exposed to a magnetic field are capable of receiving and then re-transmitting electromagnetic energy with the strength proportional to proton density. The latest form of MRI is called functional magnetic resonance imaging (fMRI), which can distinctly highlight active areas of the brain, but with relatively low resolution. In the case of both CT and MRI, a sophisticated computerized algorithm reconstructs an image of each slice.

Another technology for imaging the living brain is the positron emission topography (PET) scanner. This system uses injected radioactive labeled compounds and allows the brain's changing blood flow to be measured and recorded with relatively high resolution. The PET camera part of the system is a donut-shaped set of radioactive detectors that circle the subject's head. PET allows us to locate areas of the brain associated with specific mental operations. All of these technologies are being used by researchers to learn more about how the brain works.

The views of the brain provided by present day technologies are impressive, but the fact is that they have limited value for diagnosing brain disorders. Most diagnoses are made based on analysis of symptoms. This may change in the future as we learn more about the brain and as the capabilities and resolution of imaging devices increases. This highlights the fact that not only do we need basic brain science research, but we need the improved technology for diagnosing and treating brain disorders that such research should also produce.

It is exciting every time a significant advancement in technology is announced. For example, after 13 years of development, the National High Magnetic Field Laboratory in Tallahasee, Florida, announced the successful operation of a super conducting magnet, weighing more than 15 tons and having a magnetic field 420,000 times that of the earth's magnetic field. Researchers at the lab claim that the magnet will yield important discoveries in the fields of chemical and biomedical research, including brain scans at never before achieved resolution. This is good news showing important progress.

A very important and growing field of research is brain-machine interfacing, which is not only useful for diagnostic instruments, but for replacing damaged functions. As long as 150 years ago scientists demonstrated the electrical excitability of the motor cortex, which raised the possibility of interfacing a machine with the human brain. The field has already developed to the point where electrodes implanted in the cochlea have restored the perception of sound to some deaf individuals. Similar attempts are underway to provide images to the visual cortex and also to allow the brains of paralyzed patients to re-establish some control of lost functions.. The application for improved prosthetics (limb replacement) is also very significant. These fields are still in early stages of development, but have great potential, despite the fact that the brain was neither designed or located for either easy access or interfacing. The advancements in imaging and other technologies for conducting basic brain research will have far reaching effects on all of our lives.

Figure 9

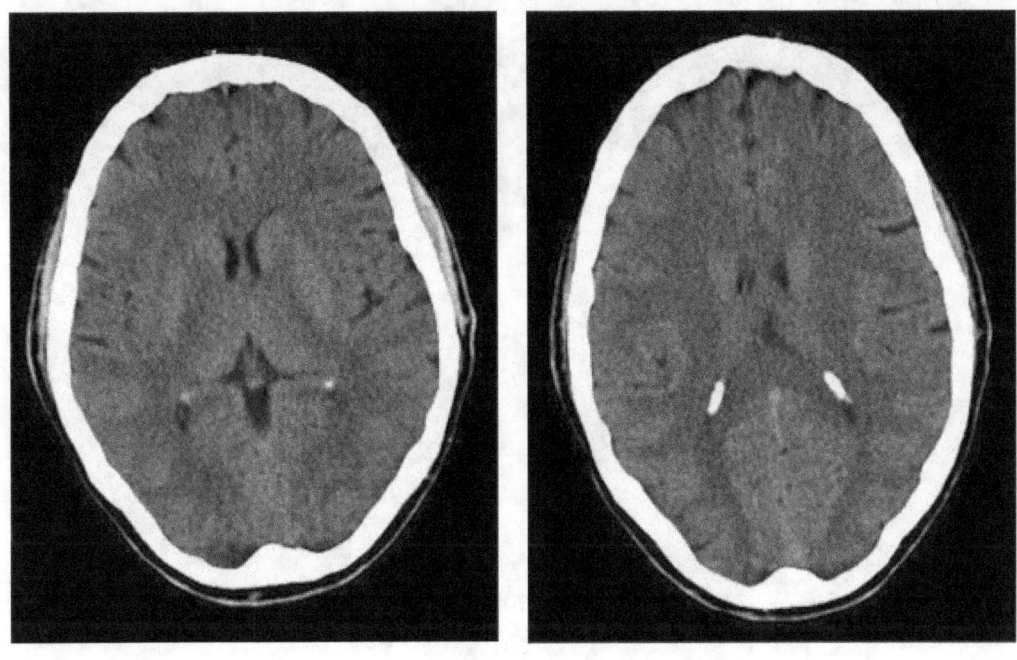

10

THE BRAIN AND THE COMPUTER

The brain and the computer are both information processors, but they differ in some significant ways. The brain, our bio-computer, is a living, constantly changing entity as opposed to the man-made computer which is a fixed configuration machine. The digital computer uses binary (ones and zeros) coding and processes information serially, one step at a time, and under the control of a master timing clock, usually operating in the GHZ (1,000,000,000 hz) frequency range. The brain processes information in parallel with many special-purpose processors. Computer systems have been built with multiple processors performing parallel processing as well. The brain's processing speed is relatively slow, below 200 HZ, because it uses a combination of bio-chemical and bio-electrical conductivity, as opposed to the purely electrical conductivity of computers. The main functional difference between the computer and the brain is that the brain can reason, think, and generate creative ideas. The brain has consciousness, the computer does not. In this sense the brain still stands alone as the premier information processor.

The brain can be considered a special purpose computer, and it clearly cannot do many things that a general purpose digital computer can do faster and more accurately. The brain is better at doing some jobs, and the computer is better at others, especially where huge amounts of data is involved. The computer follows instructions contained in software. The brain operates in accordance with its evolved architecture, and its software and hardware equivalents to the computer are not separate, and this is a fundamental difference between the brain and the computer.

Digital computers are called "digital" because their architecture is based on the binary number system which has only two digits, namely "0" and "1". These two states are created in electronic form using a switching device that can be either OFF (O) or ON (1). Remarkably, the computer uses only the numbers 0 and 1, called bits, to perform all of its calculations and processing. Every letter, number, and symbol is translated into some number of bits (32 in most modern computers) and this group of bits is called a byte. It is this multiple bit coding system that gives the computer its versatility while being based on a simple ON/OFF basic circuit element. A computer's architecture is made up of three main subdivisions, namely the central processor unit

(CPU), the memory unit, and the input/output (I/O) interface as shown in figure 10a. Two way data transmission takes place between these three major parts of the computer and also with the external world. As information processors, it is not surprising that the basic overall architecture of both the brain and the computer are somewhat similar.

The building block, or fundamental individual component of the computer is the transistor, which was developed at Bell Laboratories in the late 1940's, and led to physicist William Shockley winning a Nobel prize for his part in the development of the first silicon transistor, truly a major scientific breakthrough. The transistor, a solid-state version of its predecessor vacuum tube, made it possible for a small amount of electrical current to control a second, much stronger current, thereby performing a switching function. The switching function between "zero" or "one" states is fundamental to binary digital signal processing. Transistor switching devices are not used simply to record and manipulate numbers in computers, since the bits can just as easily stand for true (1) or not true (0), which allows computers to execute what is called Boolean algebra (logic). Combinations of transistors in various configurations are called logic gates, and these elements are combined into circuits that perform higher order processing. Computers also contain a variety of other special purpose circuits such as encoders, decoders, flip-flops, multiplexers, adders, subtractors and others. The computer is made up of many sequential sub-circuits, all synchronized by a single master clock pulse. With today's fabrication technology, many thousands (even millions) of transistors are connected on a single slice of silicon, called a chip or a microprocessor. A more recent version of the original transistor called a field-effect transistor (FET) has been replacing the conventional transistor because of its greater efficiency, which results from the fact that there is no current flow through the "gate" terminal of a FET whereas there is current flow through the "base" terminal of the bipolar transistor. The technology of computers is referred to as solid-state technology, which is much different from what could be called the "soft-state" technology of the brain. Each has its relative advantages and disadvantages.

Interestingly, both the computer and the brain are built from a basic circuit element which for the computer is the transistor, and for the brain is the neuron. Both devices are switches in the sense that they have "off" and "on" states. The neuron "on" state is temporary in that the fixed-amplitude action potential is initiated by input signals, but terminates on its own. Both devices have "thresholding" properties which provide an important measure of system noise immunity. This means that only reasonably strong signals will initiate the switching actions, which is how information is processed. This is one of the basic advantages of digital (or some switching scheme such as used in the brain) compared to pure analog (linear) signal processing, in that a high level of noise immunity is achieved. The computer's data bit is always a clock duration in width, and the repetition frequency is always the master clock frequency. The brain's data bit, the action potential is also of fixed width, but the repetition-rate is variable (from about 1-100 HZ) and this variation usually represents intensity (amplitude) information.

Neural networks are simplified models of the brain composed of large numbers of units that simulate neurons, together with weights that measure the strength of connection between units. These weights model the effects of the synapses in the brain circuitry. Experiments on models of this kind have demonstrated an ability to learn such skills as face recognition, reading, and the detection of simple grammatical structures. Neural networks are usually not built with electronic components, but are modeled on a computer. In the process of relating brain to computer functioning, we are learning more about how the brain works, so the effort is worthwhile.

During my years as an electronics systems design engineer, I saw electronics technology advance from vacuum tubes, to the individual transistor, to microchips. System designs progressed from entirely analog to mostly digital, as the digital revolution came upon us. Low-cost personal computers and a myriad of other products have resulted from the digital revolution. But it is interesting to note that both the brain and digital processors have to interface with the analog outside world. Digital systems do this with analog-to-digital and digital-to-analog converter circuitry. The brain does this by means of a variety of specialized receptors which were discussed in chapter 3.

The components in modern electronics systems are now almost entirely solid-state. Electrical signal processing is based on current flow (electrons) and use conductors and semi-conductors which are easier to fabricate and assemble in solid-structure form. This then represents one basic difference in design between the "soft-state" nature-made brain and the solid-state man-made products. Interestingly, the human body has some solid-state structures called bones, but nature apparently decided that the complexity of the information processing job of the brain required a soft-state design.

We engineers felt that we could design reliable systems that theoretically could last forever, by using solid-state design and by making the system maintainable and repairable. The latest systems have incorporated elaborate built-in-test features which allow the systems to continuously monitor performance and to identify failed hardware. One could say that the human organism has some effective built-in-test features, with the main one being our ability to feel pain, and even to predict some developing problems. Certain types of headaches (called stress or tension headaches) are probably a warning of an overworked brain. "Panic attacks" may be a built-in warning of a chronically over-worked stress-response system.

With all of the amazing progress in various technologies, we have yet to come close to producing an information processor to match the human brain. And why should we want to come up with a superior version of ourselves, assuming we could do that ? It would make us obsolete! Making ourselves obsolete would not make any sense. Technology has displaced large numbers of workers, and retraining of workers will continue to be required. Engineers will continue to improve their designs, and both computers and robots will advance in terms of tasks in which they can outperform their human counterparts. How the future will all work for human vs. machine is unclear. What is clear is that our goal as a world-wide society should be to help make the lives of all of its citizens as satisfying and productive as possible. And in order to do that we need to continue to understand exactly how the human organism works, especially the brain. As the lifespan of the human organism increases, it is interesting to think about what the maximum might be and how this might change societies. Assuming that the earth can only support some maximum number of humans, longer lifetimes would have to be balanced with birthrates. These are issues beyond science alone.

The nature-made-brain and the man-made-computer are both information processors, but as we have discussed, they represent very different design concepts. This is unfortunate with respect to cross-fertilization of knowledge. Mathematicians and engineers did get interested in the field of neural networks, but their application to digital processing systems is limited at best. More electrical engineers and physicists have to get involved in brain science research, so that they can help the biologists and chemists figure out how the brain works. Once we know more about how it works, we will be better able to figure out how best to fix problems and how we can keep our brain healthy and productive for the longest possible time.

FIGURE 10 (a) COMPUTER ARCHITECTURE

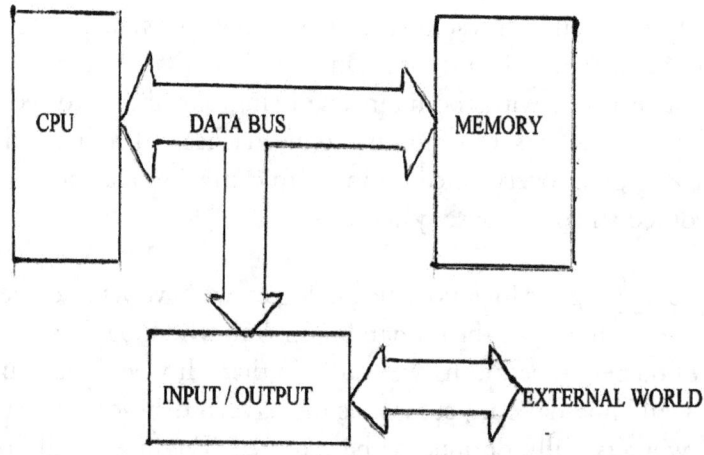

11

MYSTERIES

1. BRAIN DISORDERS

Some researchers are predicting that over half of all Americans will suffer at least one episode of some kind of serious mental illness during their lifetime. With a statistic like this, my choice for #1 brain mystery is the lack of understanding as to the exact causes of most brain disorders. To be simply told that one has a chemical imbalance in their brain, but there is no diagnostic test to prove it, and no scientific explanation for why it happened, is proof that a lot needs to be learned about the brain and mental illness. A new drug coming on the market almost every day is not proof of important advancements in neuroscience, despite the implications in the billion dollar marketing campaigns of drug companies. We need to make it more profitable for drug companies to spend this money on basic neuroscience than on advertising. Maybe it would be possible for our government to award specific research contracts to drug companies that agree to limit their marketing efforts to doctors only.

Following is a list of the more common brain disorders that still require research into cause, treatment, and hopefully prevention:

ALZHEIMER'S- The most common form of dementia.

AUTISM- A condition beginning in infancy with various degrees of mental disability, including social interaction, repetitive behaviors, and language problems.

CANCER/TUMORS- Growths either benign or malignant.

CEREBRAL PALSY- A condition in which the part of the brain causing movement does not develop properly.

DEMENTIA- A persistent loss of memory and intellectual function that is severe enough to interfere with normal life.

EPILEPSY- Abnormal electrical discharges in the brain resulting in a fit or seizure.

HYDROCEPHALUS- A build up of fluids in the ventricles of the brain causing an increase of pressure within the skull.

MENINGITIS- Inflammation of the meninges (membranes around the brain) caused by a viral or bacterial infection.

MULTIPLE SCLEROSIS- A condition that damages the nerves of the brain and spinal cord, causing various degrees of disability.

PARKINSON'S- A degeneration of the brain's basal ganglia causing muscle movement degeneration.

TAY-SACHS- An inherited condition causing a child's brain to develop abnormally, and is eventually fatal.

For a detailed description of all classes of mental illness, one should refer to the Diagnostic and Statistical Manual of Mental Disorders, fourth edition, produced by the American Psychiatric Association. This is a very readable reference book by the average person, but it does not provide information as to treatment options. The non-profit Madison Institute of Medicine, in Madison Wisconsin (www.miminc.org) is an excellent source of treatment information for mental illnesses.

We need to determine exactly how genetics and environment each contribute to brain disorders. Some neuroscientists have proposed that the prefrontal cortex, hippocampus, and amygdala are altered in some way in almost all forms of mental illness. This may be an important clue as to where to concentrate research efforts. There is in fact a lot of neuroscience research going on in America and around the world. It is not clear that America will contunue to be the leader in scientific research, as it clearly has been in the past. The number of American students pursuing careers in science and engineering will be inadequate to maintaining a leadership role in scientific research. This is a serious problem for us to work on at all levels of our educational system..

2. CONSCIOUSNESS (AWARENESS)

The most astonishing of brain mysteries is how patterns of neuronal activity in a three pound mass of jelly-like tissue become transformed into subjective awareness, consciousness, and the sense of self that all humans have. This question has puzzled scientists for ages. Neuroscientists describe four states of consciousness other than the normal conscious resting state, that include 1) deep sleep, 2) general anesthesis, 3) vegetative state or coma, and 4) epileptic loss of consciousness. All of these are considered unconscious states, and pet scans show that as compared to the conscious state, they exhibit low brain activity, especially between the thalamus and cortex, as well as different EEG waveforms. The thalamus is particularly interesting as a module in the brain that may do more than originally believed. All of the sensory information (except smell) is first routed through the thalamus before being directed to other areas of the brain for further processing. Two way connections exist between the thalamus and cortex. The thalamus is located at about the exact center of the brain, which is probably the most secure location and consistent with where one would locate a more important brain function than the relay station that it has been traditionally believed to be. It seems logical that somewhere in the brain there has to be output transducers of some type that create in us the sensations of seeing, hearing, etc. These output transducers might contain some form of digital to analog converter to transform the neurons frequency modulated pulse signals to an analog signal. For now this process remains a very challenging mystery.

Consciousness has been described as the end result of information processing occurring unconsciously. Another way to think about consciousness is to consider it an awareness of what is in working (short-term) memory. Clearly without memory, there could be no consciousness. Do any other animals have a self-awareness? No one knows for sure.

3. MEMORY

One important question for brain science to answer is how memory works and exactly where in the brain are memories stored. There does not appear to be a single location for all memory, and we have both a short-term and a long-term memory. There appears to be a special memory capability in the limbic (stress response) section of the brain in order to allow rapid response to threats, while the thinking portion (cortex) considers longer-term responses. Other special memory ability for learned movements apparently resides in the cerebellum (which is near the brain-stem) and is our movement controller. It is capable of storing learned physical activity such as walking, riding a bicycle, etc. The main location for our short and long term memory is believed to be in the cortex.

Traumatic event memories seem to be handled differently than other memories. These types of memories or other emotional events remain unusually stable over time. Traumatic and emotional memories are believed to be stored by the hippocampus (of the limbic system), which organizes the information and integrates it with previous memories of similar sensory details. The amygdala (also part of the limbic system) attaches emotional significance to the sensory information and passes it on to the hippocampus for storage.

The synaptic theory of memory was mentioned in chapter 7, and is the one most neuroscientists seem to have embraced. The ability to remember is fundamental to being alive. It is the central ability of the brain that pulls together learning, understanding, and consciousness. It appears that the hippocampus might perform the function of master regulator for memories. Without it one cannot learn or remember anything. But it is not believed to be the place where all memories are stored. Recent research indicates that sleep may play a role in recording memories. It appears that REM sleep in particular is involved with organizing pieces, and the association between them, needed to form lasting memories. Learning and memory processes are closely linked. Learning enables information to cross the lines of perception into memory.

As mentioned before, we have both short-term and long-term memory. The former lasts for minutes or hours, and the latter for more than a day. Short-term memory is sometimes called working memory, which in the computer is called random-access-memory (RAM), which holds data we are working with, but loses it when no longer needed or the power is turned off. Long-term memory is like the computer's hard disk, which retains data for as long as we desire. When we learn the exact mechanism in the brain for memory storage, we may then be able to prevent the memory loss that is associated with certain brain disorders, and this understanding will also be important to education. No one knows what the brain's memory capacity is, although there must be some physical limitation. It may be that as one's memory capacity is reached that new memories simply displace certain old memories. A better understanding of how memory works will have important application to educational methods.

4. SLEEP

We spend almost 1/3 of our lives sleeping, therefore one would conclude that it may be more important than might appear. The exact purposes of sleep remain one of the important mysteries of neuroscience. The pineal gland located deep within the brain appears to be our biological clock, and secretes melatonin, a sleep related hormone that effects brain cells that use the neurotransmitter seratonin. Various stages of sleep have been identified, with dreaming occurring during the REM (rapid eye movement) stage, which is the one closest to wakefulness. During sleep the cortex is in the unaroused state, except during dream (REM) sleep when it is highly aroused, except that it is only processing internal information. The possible function of dreaming is also a mystery associated with sleeping. Sleep disorders are a problem for a relatively large portion of the population (about 10 %), and can lead to more serious illnesses.

Surely most of us have had the experience of waking up with a new idea or a solution to one of yesterday's problems. This would seem to indicate that we are doing more than just "recharging our batteries" while asleep. The brain seems to be taking full advantage of this down time by sending some information to the recycle bin, while retaining and even refining some of the filtered out data. Without the virtual flood of incoming sensory data, the brain is apparently free for other housekeeping and even creative chores. But how much sleep does each of us really need? Is there a physiological difference between waking up with an alarm clock compared to natural wake-up? What things will help to optimize our time spent sleeping? Researchers are working to learn more about these and many more questions about the relatively large percentage of our lives we spend in the mind-altered state called sleep.

5. BRAIN WIRING DIAGRAM (SCHEMATIC)

Another unknown is exactly how the brain is wired. The brain seems to be a configuration of many special purpose processors working in parallel, but with many interconnections between them as well. Neuronal type networks have been studied by mathematicians and scientists and have been shown to perform processing functions such as those believed to be performed by the brain. But mapping of actual brain circuitry has yet to be accomplished. We know a lot about the basic electrical and chemical functioning of the brain, but the actual interconnection configuration remains a mystery.

No one could understand or effectively work on a complex man-made electronics system without having a detailed schematic showing how the individual components are interconnected into circuits and then larger assemblies. This should be one of the highest priorities for neuroscientists. The field of neural networks seems to have become separated from basic neuroscience, possibly because they involve different specialties. But they will need to work together to generate a detailed and accurate schematic of the typical brain.

We know that the brain processes information using a massive number of neurons arrayed in parallel, specialized processor networks. In addition to not knowing how the neurons are wired into circuits, we also don't know exactly how the information is coded. The structure of the neural code has been a fundamental question in systems neuroscience for almost a century. Certain theories have been proposed but experimental data to prove their validity is yet to be obtained. From my very limited study of the literature it seems that the coding scheme is related to a form of digital (binary) signal processing, with pulse frequency modulation, but the brain's circuit (network) configurations also have some analog signal processing characteristics, such as feedback loops, dendrite summation circuitry, and variable threshold controls. Is it possible that the designer of the brain used a combination of the best of all techniques?

6. GENETICS AND ENVIRONMENT

The age old question of nature vs. nurture applies to the brain. We need to know the exact contributions of genetics and environment. Understanding the role of genetics will be a strong factor in being able to prevent and hopefully cure conditions that are strongly under genetic control. We clearly are not a product of our genes alone, and we learn more and more every day about the importance of diet and exercise to optimum health (for the brain and the rest of the body). However, what constitutes an optimal diet? The traditional medical and the alternative medicine communities have been in disagreement over this question for years. There is no consensus as to the real value of dietary supplements either. These questions need scientific answers. Other environmental factors such as the air that we breath, and other toxins we are exposed to, also need to remain a high priority for study and control

7. GLIA CELLS

Glia cells outnumber neurons by about 10 to 1. The exact functions of these cells is still not well understood, and this area of study may reveal important new information about the overall brain works.

My purpose in this chapter was to highlight the fact that many fundamental questions about the brain remain to be answered. This list is certainly not all-inclusive, and I would challenge the neuroscience community to publish their own list, and not leave the impression that the search for new drug treatments for mental illness is the only challenge.

SUMMARY

It may be useful to connect the field of brain science with the fields of information technology, engineering, and physics, so as to elevate it beyond the interest of medical science alone. Medical science is strongly bio-chemistry oriented and not strong in physics or engineering. As we know, the brain is very much electrical and even mechanical, and these are specialties that most medical researchers do not have. The engineering community has been involved in the bio-medical field, but primarily in terms of developing instrumentation technology. This situation needs to change if we want to accelerate the advancement of brain science.

Most people recognize that exploring "outer space" is in the long-term best interests of the human race and we are devoting considerable resources to this effort. I approve of the exploration of space because of the many already achieved and potential benefits, but my preference would be to postpone manned exploration and emphasize unmanned, robotic missions. The costs in dollars and lives would be much lower, and the robotics technology advancements would have both military and civilian application. The cross-fertilization between neuroscience and robotics science could be significant. But the most important point here is that we need the same kind of national commitment to adequately funded, goal oriented, exploration of inner-space as we have for outer-space. Public relations efforts such as announcing "The Decade of the Brain", in the 1990's is evidence that our policy-makers do not understand the scope of the job involved, or the relative importance of doing this basic neuroscience research. Many well-respected scientists believe the task of unlocking the brain's secrets may be equivalent to the challenge of unlocking the secrets of the universe. But significant progress has and is continuing to be made in neuroscience research, and the prospects for advancements in the future are significant, and these discoveries will change the course of human evolution.

Many like to characterize the present as the information age. One could argue that the information age started with the evolution of the human species, which happened to include the world's first information processor, the human brain. But we now need a national, high-priority program for the exploration of inner space, which would need to include new technology development needed to explore the sub-microscopic world. It will take this new technology to eventually map the human brain and attempt to un-lock its remaining secrets. In the process we will be able to learn how to more effectively treat and even prevent brain disorders, as well as to improve public education methods. Recent studies have indicated that 50% of Americans will experience some category of mental illness in their lifetimes. This alone should be a strong motivator for accelerated research in the field of brain science.

The combination of electronics technology and neuroscience advancements has almost unlimited potential for benefits in the treatment of some brain disorders. Early results in the improvement of hearing and sight problems are already encouraging.

As far as we know the human brain has not physically changed significantly for many thousands of years. The human condition, however, has changed quite dramatically. Was the human brain designed for this kind of flexibility and adaptability? Only time will tell. The capacity of the human brain is being tested by time, and this is probably the methodology of evolution. The difference in this case is that we may be the masters of our own fate, with respect to how we use our brains. The basic tool that we have for unlocking the remaining unknowns about the brain is the brain itself. Is it up to the task? Fortunately, scientists are always motivated by challenging questions, and very many talented people are presently working to unlock the remaining secrets of the human brain. We can all do our part in promoting this important work by urging our government officials to place a higher national priority on this work, keep the effort goal-oriented, and provide adequate funding. This task is far beyond just a medical issue, and it is reasonable to suggest that a positive future course of history will depend on unlocking the remaining secrets of the human brain.

Educators report that students embrace neuroscience topics with great enthusiasm, and are eager to learn more about themselves. Science in general and neuroscience in particular are great ways for children to learn how to learn. If we think of neuroscience as a frontier, we can appreciate the benefits of attracting capable students to careers in this exciting and critical career.

REFERENCES

Abdi, Valentin, & Edelman, "Neural Networks", Sage Publications 1999

Andreasen, Nancy C. M.D., PhD. "The Broken Brain" New York, Harper & Row 1984.

Andreasen, Nancy C. M.D., PhD. " Brave New Brain" New York, Oxford University Press 2001.

Averbeck, B. & Lee, D. (2004) Coding and transmission of information by neural assemblies. Trends in Neuroscience Vol. 27 No. 4

Baars, B. Ramsey, T. and Laureys, S. (2003) Brain, conscious experience and the observing self. Trends in Neuroscience Vol. 26 No. 12

Beck, Aaron T. M.D. "Cognitive Therapy and The Emotional Disorders" Connecticut, Meridian 1976.

Diagnostic and Statistical Manual of Mental Disorders, Fourth Edition, Text Revision (DSM-IV-TR), Washington D.C. American Psychiatric Association 2000.

Greenfield, Susan. "Brain Story" London, BBC Worldwide 2000

Guttman, Griffiths, Suzuki, Cullis. "Genetics- A Beginner's Guide" Oxford, England, Oneworld Publications 2002

Huxley, Andrew (2002) From overshoot to voltage clamp. Trends in Neuroscience Vol. 25 No. 11

Johnson, Steven. "Mind Wide Open" New York, Scribner 2004

LeDoux, Joseph "The Emotional Brain" New York. Touchstone Books 1998

LeDoux, Joseph "Synaptic Self" New York. Penguin Books 2002

Madison Institute of Medicine, Madison Wisconsin (608) 827-2470 www.mimic.org

McEwen, Bruce "The End of Stress As We Know It" Washington D.C. Joseph Henry Press 2002

McFadden, Johnjoe. "Quantum Evolution" New York, W.W. Norton & Company 2000

Meunier, C. & Segev, I. (2002) Playing the devil's advocate: Is the Hodgkin-Huxley model useful? Trends in Neuroscience Vol. 25 No. 11

NARSAD Research Newsletters.

Longstaff, A. "Neuroscience" Oxford, U.K. Bios Publishers 2000

Piccolino, Marco (2002) Fifty years of the Hodgkin-Huxley era. Trends in Neuroscience. Vol. 25 No. 11

Pinker, Steven "How the Mind Works" New York, W.W. Norton & Co.1997

Posner and Raichle "Images of Mind" Scientific American Library, New York 1999

Ratey, John J. M.D. "A User's Guide to the Brain" New York, Scribner 2004

Restak, Richard M.D. "The Secret Life of the Brain" Washington D.C. Joseph Henry Press 2001

Restak. Richard M.D. "Mysteries of the Mind" National Geographic, Wash. D.C. 2000

Sapolsky, Robert M. "Why Zebras Don't Get Ulcers" New York. W.H. Freeman & Co. 1998

Satinover, Jeffrey "The Quantum Brain" New York, John Wiley & Sons 2001

Schwartz, Jeffrey M. M.D. "The Mind and the Brain", New York, Regan Books 2002

Shanor, Karen Nesbitt "The Emerging Mind" Los Angeles. Rennaissance Books 1999

Society for Neuroscience, "Brain Facts" (2002)

Tsay, D. & Yuste, R. (2004) On the electrical function of dendritic spines. Trends in Neuroscience Vol. 27 No. 2

Turkington, Carol. "The Brain Encyclopedia" New York/ Checkmark Books 1996

Victoroff, Jeff M.D. "Saving Your Brain" New York. Bantam Books 2002

WEB SITES: all start with www.

brain science.brown.edu

klab.caltech.edu

sciencedirect.com

questia.com

nature.com

hhmi.org

willamette.edu

unm.edu

uni.edu

bioweb.uncc.edu

sfn.org

synapses.mcg.edu

whatislife.com

sky.bsd.Chicago.edu

online-medical-dictionary.org

indstate.edu

rei.Rutgers.edur

neurosci.pharm.utoledo.edu

chemistry.emory.edu

pubs.acs.org

med.Harvard.edu

ABOUT THE AUTHOR

Mr. Amoroso has a bachelor degree in electrical engineering and a master degree in business administration and is retired from a 30 year career with a major aerospace company. During his career he had both electronics systems design and technical management experience with participation in all phases of diversified, high-technology radar and communications development programs. He has 12 patents granted in the areas of microwave radar and communications. His career spanned the eras of vacuum tubes, individual transistors, and integrated circuits, and from almost entirely analog designs to combinations of analog and digital systems design. Since retiring, his new passion has become learning as much as possible about how the central processing unit (CPU) of the body, called the brain, really works. He has recently formed an organization called Brain Research Advocates Information Network (B.R.A.I.N.) in order to spread the word about the challenges, benefits of, and progress in basic neuroscience research. Address correspondence to;

Salvatore Amoroso
2303 89th St NW
Bradenton, Fl 34209
E-mail address:
samoroso@tampabay.rr.com

www.ingramcontent.com/pod-product-compliance
Lightning Source LLC
Chambersburg PA
CBHW081217170526
45165CB00009B/2850